Thyroid For Dumm...

MW00338329

Maximising Your Thyroid Health

For more information about these steps, see Chapter 21:

- If thyroid disease runs in your family, ask your doctor about screening for thyroid diseases at appropriate intervals.

- If you have a thyroid problem, check your thyroid function during times of major body changes, such as pregnancy.

- Make sure you get enough iodine in your diet, especially if you are a vegetarian.

- If you've taken thyroid hormone replacement for several years to treat hypothyroidism (low thyroid function), ask your doctor if you can try stopping treatment to see if your thyroid can function without it.

- If you still experience symptoms of hypothyroidism while taking hormone replacement pills, ask your doctor if you can try taking both types of thyroid hormone (T4 and T3), although this is controversial.

- Remember that some medications can interact with thyroid hormones. (For a complete discussion of drug interactions, see Chapter 10.)

- Protect your thyroid from radiation. If your neck has had exposure to radiation in the past, ensure your doctor knows that.

- Remember that new discoveries regularly occur in thyroid health and treatment. Appendix B features many Web sites that help you keep up to date.

Signs and Symptoms of Low Thyroid Function

Someone with hypothyroidism – an under-active thyroid gland – often experiences some of the following signs and symptoms. (Keep in mind that these symptoms alone can't diagnose thyroid disease, and thyroid disease is sometimes present even if you don't experience all these symptoms. See Chapter 5 for detailed information about hypothyroidism.)

- Slow pulse
- Enlarged thyroid (unless removed during previous thyroid treatment)
- Dry, cool skin that is puffy, pale, and yellowish
- Brittle nails and dry, brittle hair that falls out excessively
- Swelling, especially of the legs
- Hoarseness, slow speech, and a thickened tongue
- Slow reflexes
- Intolerance to cold
- Tiredness and a need to sleep excessively
- Constipation
- Increased menstrual flow

For Dummies: Bestselling Book Series for Beginners

Thyroid For Dummies®

Cheat Sheet

Signs and Symptoms of Excessive Thyroid Function

Someone with hyperthyroidism – an over-active thyroid gland – may experience some or all of the following symptoms. (The same caution about symptoms of hypothyroidism applies here; these symptoms alone don't confirm a diagnosis. Only blood tests can do this. See Chapter 6 for more information about hyperthyroidism.)

- Higher body temperature and intolerance to heat
- Weight loss
- Weakness
- Enlarged thyroid
- Warm, moist skin
- Rapid pulse
- Tremor of the fingers and tongue
- Nervousness
- Difficulty sleeping
- Rapid mood changes
- Decreased menstrual flow
- More frequent bowel movements
- Changes to the eyes that make it appear as if you're staring

Medications to Watch Out For

Certain drugs can interact with your thyroid hormone to negatively affect your thyroid function. Chapter 10 goes into detail about this subject, but these are just a few commonly used medications that can affect your thyroid:

- Amiodarone
- Aspirin (more than 3,000 milligrams daily)
- Oestrogen (for example, in hormone replacement therapy, or in the oral contraceptive pill)
- Iron tablets
- Iodine
- Lithium
- Propranolol
- Corticosteroids

For Dummies: Bestselling Book Series for Beginners

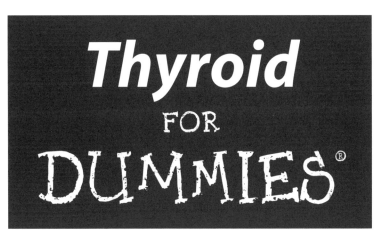

Thyroid
FOR
DUMMIES®

by
Alan L. Rubin, MD
Dr Sarah Brewer

John Wiley & Sons, Ltd

Thyroid For Dummies®

Published by
John Wiley & Sons, Ltd
The Atrium
Southern Gate
Chichester
West Sussex
PO19 8SQ
England

E-mail (for orders and customer service enquires): cs-books@wiley.co.uk

Visit our Home Page on www.wiley.com

For general information on our other products and services, please contact our Customer Care Department within the U.S. at 800-762-2974, outside the U.S. at 317-572-3993, or fax 317-572-4002.

For technical support, please visit www.wiley.com/techsupport.

Wiley also publishes its books in a variety of electronic formats. Some content that appears in print may not be available in electronic books.

British Library Cataloguing in Publication Data: A catalogue record for this book is available from the British Library

ISBN-13: 978-0-470-03172-8

ISBN-10: 0-470-03172-7

Printed and bound in Great Britain by Bell & Bain Ltd, Glasgow

10 9 8 7 6 5 4 3 2 1

About the Authors

Dr Sarah Brewer qualified as a doctor in 1983 from Cambridge University. She was a full-time GP for five years and now works in nutritional medicine and sexual health. Sarah is currently completing an MSc in Nutritional Medicine at the University of Surrey, Guildford.

Although her first love is medicine, her major passion is writing. Sarah writes widely on all aspects of health and has written over 40 popular self-help books. She is a regular contributor to a number of newspapers and women's magazines, and appears regularly on TV and radio. She was voted Health Journalist of the Year 2002.

Alan L. Rubin, MD, is one of the US's foremost experts on the thyroid gland in health and disease. He is a member of the Endocrine Society and has been in private practice specialising in thyroid disease and diabetes for over 30 years. Dr. Rubin was Assistant Clinical Professor of Medicine at UC Medical Center in San Francisco for 20 years. He has spoken about the thyroid to professional medical audiences and non-medical audiences around the world. He is a consultant to many pharmaceutical companies and companies that make thyroid products.

Dr. Rubin has written extensively on the thyroid gland as well as diabetes mellitus. As a result, he has been on numerous radio and television programs, talking about the cause, the prevention, and the treatment of conditions of the thyroid. He is also the best-selling author of *Diabetes For Dummies* and *Diabetes Cookbook For Dummies*.

Dedication

From Alan: This book is dedicated to my wife, Enid, who was there for every page. She smilingly let me do my work, sometimes into the wee hours of the morning, and missed many an opportunity to go out to dinner or a movie so that I could produce this book for you. If you have a fraction of the support in your life that she has given me, you are a lucky person, indeed.

Authors' Acknowledgements

From Alan: The great publisher and midwife, Kathy Nebenhaus, deserves enormous appreciation for helping me to deliver yet another bright-eyed baby. Her optimism and her enthusiasm actually made this book possible. Her assistant, Natasha Graf, played a huge role in ironing out the inevitable problems that arise when book-publishing and medicine meet.

My editor, Joan Friedman, did a magnificent job turning my sometimes-incomprehensible prose into words that you can understand. She also conducted a whole orchestra of other editors who contributed to the book, including Robert Annis, Christy Beck, Mary Fales, Alison Jefferson, and Greg Pearson.

My thanks to Dr. Catherine Bain for the technical editing of the book.

Librarians Mary Ann Zaremska and Nancy Phelps at St. Francis Memorial Hospital were tremendously helpful in providing the articles and books upon which the information in this book is based.

My teachers are too numerous to mention, but one person deserves special attention. Dr. Francis Greenspan at the University of California Medical Center gave me the sound foundation in thyroid function and disease upon which this book is based.

Finally, there are my patients over the last 28 years, the people whose trials and tribulations caused me to seek the knowledge that you will find in this book.

This book is written on the shoulders of thousands of men and women who made the discoveries, tried the medications, and held the committee meetings. Their accomplishments cannot possibly be given adequate acclaim. We owe them big time.

From Sarah: Thanks to Alan L. Rubin, MD, author of the original US version of *Thyroid For Dummies*. The quality of his original script made my job easy, as I had so very little to do when adapting his excellent book for the UK market.

Publisher's Acknowledgements

We're proud of this book; please send us your comments through our Dummies online registration form located at www.dummies.com/register/.

Some of the people who helped bring this book to market include the following:

Acquisitions, Editorial, and Media Development

Commissioning Editor: Alison Yates

Project Editor: Simon Bell

Copy Editor: Juliet Booker

Technical Editor: Georges Mouton

Executive Editor: Jason Dunne

Executive Project Editor: Martin Tribe

Cover Photo: GettyImages/Marc Romanelli

Cartoons: Ed McLachlan

Composition Services

Project Coordinator: Jennifer Theriot

Layout and Graphics: Claudia Bell, Carl Byers, Denny Hager, LeAndra Hosier, Lynsey Osborn

Proofreader: Susan Moritz

Indexer: Techbooks

Special Help

Brand Reviewer: Zoe Wykes

Publishing and Editorial for Consumer Dummies

Diane Graves Steele, Vice President and Publisher, Consumer Dummies

Joyce Pepple, Acquisitions Director, Consumer Dummies

Kristin A. Cocks, Product Development Director, Consumer Dummies

Michael Spring, Vice President and Publisher, Travel

Kelly Regan, Editorial Director, Travel

Publishing for Technology Dummies

Andy Cummings, Vice President and Publisher, Dummies Technology/General User

Composition Services

Gerry Fahey, Vice President of Production Services

Debbie Stailey, Director of Composition Services

Contents at a Glance

Table of Contents

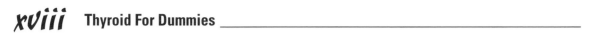

Introduction

. . . .

*A*s part of my medical training, I (Sarah) was taught by an enlightened physician, Dr David Rubenstein of Addenbrooke's Hospital, Cambridge. He encouraged me to do three things when evaluating a patient with puzzling symptoms: Think Drugs (so as not to miss unsuspected side effects), Think Dirty (to exclude syphilis, a disease that mimics so many other conditions) and Think Thyroid – because under and overactive thyroid problems are so often missed, especially in older people.

I went on to make a career out of thinking drugs and thinking thyroid (thinking dirty is no longer as necessary as it was just a generation ago).

For hundreds of years, people understood that a connection exists between a strange looking growth in the neck and certain diseases. Until about 60 years ago, confusion reigned as people with similar growths in their necks often have opposite symptoms. One group shows excessive excitement, nervousness, and shakiness, while the other has depression, sleepiness, and general loss of interest. What the two groups have in common is that they are mostly all women.

As recently as 60 years ago, scientists started to measure the chemicals coming from these growths (enlarged thyroid glands), and suddenly the whole picture began making sense. Now, many of the secrets of the thyroid gland and the hormones it makes are known, although it undoubtedly still has a few surprises up its sleeve.

This book explains that, with very rare exceptions, thyroid diseases, including thyroid cancer, are some of the most easily treated of all disorders. This fact is why many thyroid specialists say, 'If I have to have cancer, let's hope it's a thyroid cancer.'

This book reveals the thyroid in all its glory. As it regulates body temperature, one of the main symptoms of thyroid problems is feeling hot or feeling cold. Unfortunately, this symptom leads to a lot of confusion within the thyroid itself. So much so that the left lobe of the thyroid was once heard to say to the right lobe: 'Now I know it's summer – here comes another swallow.'

About This Book

The good news is that you don't need to read this book from cover to cover. Since the first few chapters are a general introduction to the thyroid, you may find it helpful to start in Part I, but if you prefer to go right to information about the thyroid condition that affects you, off you go to find it. If you run across any terms you don't understand, look for them in the glossary of terms in Appendix A.

This book is written as a sort of medical biography of a family – Toni, Stacy, Linda, Ken, and other members of the clan whom you meet during your reading. These folks illustrate the fact that thyroid disease often runs in families. You meet members of the family, as well as some other fine fictional characters, at the beginning of each chapter that describes a thyroid disease, so you have a good picture of the condition covered in that chapter.

Conventions Used in This Book

Although books such as this are easiest to read if they only use non-scientific terms, you and your doctor would soon find that you're speaking two different languages. Therefore, *Thyroid For Dummies* does use scientific terms, but these terms are explained in everyday English the first time you run across them. Plus, definitions of those difficult terms are available in the Glossary at the back of the book.

Three scientific terms come up over and over again in this book: thyroxine, triiodothyronine, and thyroid-stimulating hormone (also known as thyrotropin). These terms are explained in detail in Chapter 3. For these three words, abbreviations are used for easier reading: Thyroxine is T4, triiodothyronine is T3, and thyroid-stimulating hormone is TSH.

What You Don't Have to Read

Throughout the book, you find shaded boxes of text called sidebars. These contain interesting material but not essential to your understanding. If you don't care to go so deeply into a subject, skip the sidebars; you can still understand everything else.

Assumptions

This book assumes that you or someone you care about has a thyroid condition that is not yet treated or perhaps is not treated to your satisfaction. If this assumption doesn't apply to you, perhaps you suspect that you have a thyroid condition and want to determine whether you should see a doctor. Or perhaps you can't get your doctor to run the necessary tests to determine whether a thyroid problem exists. Regardless of your individual situation, this book has valuable information for you.

The material in the chapters does not make any assumptions about what you know regarding the thyroid and doesn't introduce any new terms without explaining what they are. If you already know a lot about the thyroid and its functions, you can still find new information that adds to your knowledge.

How This Book Is Organised

The book is divided into six parts to help you find out all you want to know about the thyroid gland.

Part I: Understanding Your Thyroid

So much (right and wrong) is written about the way the thyroid affects your mood that this issue is cleared up at the very beginning of the book. After you understand how the thyroid affects your emotions, you find out just what the thyroid is and what it does. Finally, in this part you learn about the medical tests that help to determine if something is wrong with your thyroid.

Part II: Treating Thyroid Problems

This part explains each of the conditions that affect the thyroid and how they affect you. After finishing this part of the book, you will know just about everything we know about thyroid disease, how to identify it, and how to treat it.

Part III: Managing Your Thyroid

Here you discover how medications can influence your thyroid function. We also explain thyroid infections, along with the worldwide problem of iodine deficiency. I also show you why thyroid surgery is rarely done, and look at new treatments coming along. The final two chapters look at ways to improve your thyroid health – and your health in general – using diet, exercise, lifestyle choices, and complementary therapies.

Part IV: Considering Special Aspects of Thyroid Health

Thyroid problems often run in families and this part looks at the genetic basis of some thyroid diseases. Three groups of people also deserve special consideration in this book: pregnant women, children, and those over the age of 65 years. Thyroid conditions take unusual directions in these groups, so the chapters in this part address their unique difficulties.

Part V: The Part of Tens

Misinformation about the thyroid is rampant. This part aims to clear up some of that misinformation – though not all, as it accumulates faster than dust. The information also shows you how you can maximise your thyroid health.

Part VI: Appendices

In Appendix A, you find a glossary of medical terms that relate to the thyroid; you may want to bookmark it so you can go back and forth with ease as you read other chapters. Appendix B directs you to the best-of-the-best Web sites where you can get dependable facts to fill in any blank spots that remain after you've read this book.

Icons Used in This Book

Books in the *For Dummies* series feature icons in the margins, which direct you towards information that may be of particular interest or importance. Here's an explanation of what each icon in this book signifies:

When you see this icon, it means the information is essential. You want to ensure that you understand it.

This icon points out important information that can save you time and energy.

You find this icon next to paragraphs about the family members or other folks with specific thyroid conditions.

This icon alerts you to situations in which you may need to contact your doctor for some help.

This icon warns against potential problems you could encounter, such as the side effects of mixing medications.

This icon shows where medical terms are defined.

Where to Go from Here

Where you go from here depends upon your needs. If you want to understand how the thyroid works, head to Part I. If you or someone you know has a thyroid condition, you may want to pay particular attention to Part II. For help in maintaining good thyroid health, turn to Part III. If thyroid disease runs in your family, or if you're pregnant or have a child or parent with a thyroid disorder, Part IV is your next stop. In any case, as my mother used to say when she gave me a present, use this book in good health.

Part I
Understanding the Thyroid

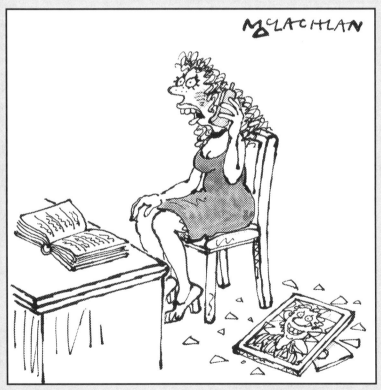

"When he said he'd got trembling hands,
rapid heartbeat, and was breaking out into a
nervous sweat, I thought it was love—then he
just said it was a thyroid problem!"

In this part . . .

What, exactly, is the thyroid gland, and what does it do? In this part, you discover how important this little gland in your neck really is, what function it plays in your body, and how to determine if it is functioning properly. We show you that your thyroid affects your mind as well as your body in critical ways.

Chapter 1

Bigging It Up: The Huge Role of a Little Gland

*Y*our thyroid is a little like Victor Meldrew, who often doesn't get the respect he feels he deserves. Anyone who watches prime-time TV knows the importance of other body parts – the heart, lungs, and wedding tackle sure get a lot of press. But unless you come face-to-face with a thyroid problem, chances are you don't hear much about what this little gland does and its vital importance to good health.

The fact that you're reading these words suggests you've encountered a thyroid problem personally. Perhaps you've recently had a thyroid condition diagnosed. Or maybe your husband, wife, mother, or friend is receiving treatment for a thyroid problem. If so, you've probably found out at least a little about this mysterious gland, and now you're looking for answers to the obvious questions that keep popping up in your mind:

✔ What causes this condition?

✔ What types of symptoms are related to this problem?

✔ How is this condition treated?

✔ What are the consequences of leaving it untreated?

✔ Does treatment end the problem forever?

✔ What can I (or my husband, wife, mother, or friend) do to help get back to optimal health?

This book aims to answer most of your questions. As doctors and researchers are constantly discovering new things about the thyroid, however, the information here is only as complete as our current knowledge. But if you're looking for concrete information about how the thyroid functions, and what to do when a problem occurs, you're holding the right paperback.

Discovering the Extent of the Problem

Thyroid disease – which is the collective term used for medical disorders of the thyroid, the majority of which are covered in this book – is one of the most common conditions in the world. Research indicates that thyroid disease affects more than 200 million people around the globe. In the United Kingdom alone, an estimated 4.5 million people have a thyroid problem out of a population of around 60.5 million. And that's just the ones who are properly diagnosed; a further two million people are believed to have over or underactive thyroid glands that remain unrecognised, although these cases are often mild.

The *incidence* of thyroid disease (the number of new cases identified annually) becomes even higher when careful autopsies are carried out on people who did not die of a thyroid condition. As many as 60 per cent of the people autopsied are found to have growths on the thyroid, and 17 per cent have small areas of cancer that were not detected during life.

These numbers are statistics, but thyroid disease affects individuals. You'll be encouraged to know that many people in the public eye have gone on to great accomplishments after being treated successfully for thyroid conditions. Some of the people you may recognise include:

- Olympic gold medal-winning sprinter, Gail Devers, had hyperthyroidism, while runner Carl Lewis had hypothyroidism.
- Author Isaac Asimov had thyroid cancer at the age of 52 and went on to live a further 20 years, eventually dying at the age of 72 from unrelated causes.
- Singer Rod Stewart had surgery to remove a thyroid growth.
- World-class golfer Ben Crenshaw had hyperthyroidism.
- Former United States President George Bush, former first lady Barbara Bush, and even their dog Millie, had hyperthyroidism – an unusual clustering that prompted extensive investigation of their water supply, although no cause was ever found.

While this list is far from exhaustive, it helps to drive home the point that, if diagnosed and treated, thyroid conditions don't need to hamper your lifestyle.

Identifying an Unhappy Thyroid

Getting down to basics, your thyroid gland lives just below your Adam's apple, at the front of your neck. (Chapter 3 gives a more detailed explanation of how to find your thyroid.) If your thyroid becomes visible in your neck, if that area of your neck is tender, or if you have some trouble swallowing or breathing, consider visiting your doctor for a thyroid checkup. Any change in the size or shape of your thyroid may mean it's not functioning properly, while soreness or tenderness can mean you have an infection or inflammation (see Chapter 11). Sometimes, a thyroid develops a growth called a *nodule,* which despite its benign sounding name is always tested to rule out cancer (see Chapter 7).

As well as changes in the size and shape of the gland, people with a malfunctioning thyroid usually develop other associated symptoms.

- ✔ If your thyroid becomes underactive, a condition known as *hypothyroidism,* you tend to put on weight, feel cold, tired, slow down, and often a little depressed. Although this description doesn't sound very specific, and these symptoms can indicate any number of other physical problems, an underactive thyroid gland is a common enough cause to ask your doctor to check things out, especially if you are over the age of 35. Chapter 5 gives you the specifics about the causes and symptoms of hypothyroidism.

- ✔ If your thyroid function is too high, a condition known as *hyperthyroidism,* you may lose weight, feel hyper and warm, and notice that your heart tends to race. You may have trouble sitting still, and your emotions may change very rapidly for no clear reason. These symptoms are a little more specific than those for low thyroid function, but again, they can easily result from some cause not related to your thyroid. Chapter 6 offers a detailed look at hyperthyroidism.

The best way to determine whether a thyroid problem exists is to ask your doctor to check your thyroid function.

Recognising Who's at Risk

A few key facts help doctors determine whether thyroid disease is a strong possibility for a given patient:

- ✔ Thyroid problems are around ten times more frequent in women than men.
- ✔ Thyroid conditions tend to run in families.
- ✔ Thyroid problems often arise after the age of 30.

These findings don't mean that a 20-year-old man with no family history of thyroid problems can't develop a thyroid condition. They simply suggest that a 35-year-old woman whose mother was diagnosed with low thyroid function 20 years ago is at greater risk of having a thyroid problem than a young male. With this in mind, any young woman with a similar family history is wise to inform her doctor, as her GP is likely to test her periodically to ensure her thyroid function is normal.

Realising the Importance of a Healthy Thyroid

Your thyroid gland influences almost every cell and organ in your body because its main function is to regulate your metabolism. If your thyroid is functioning correctly, your *metabolic rate* (the amount of energy your body burns while resting) is normal. If your thyroid is working too hard, your metabolism is too high, and you may notice an increased body temperature or an elevated heart rate. When your thyroid function drops below normal, so does your metabolism; you may gain weight, feel tired, and experience digestive problems.

Chapter 3 details how your thyroid affects various parts of your body – in fact, just about everything – including your muscles, heart, lungs, stomach, intestines, skin, hair, nails, brain, bones, and sexual organs.

As if that weren't enough, the thyroid also affects your mental health. People with an underactive thyroid often experience depression, while those with thyroids that work too hard are often anxious, jittery, irritable, and unable to concentrate. The mental and emotional consequences of a thyroid problem are so important and so often misunderstood that Chapter 2 is devoted to exploring and explaining these topics.

Treating What Ails You

Depending on the specific thyroid problem you're suffering from, your treatment options can range from taking a daily pill to having surgery to remove part or all of your thyroid gland.

- **Underactive thyroid.** In the United Kingdom, many GPs manage the treatment of an underactive thyroid gland on their own. You may not need to see a specialist if your condition is well controlled.

- **Overactive thyroid.** A patient with an overactive thyroid gland is ideally referred to an *endocrinologist,* a specialist who dabbles daily in different hormone problems. If your symptoms are causing difficulty while you're waiting to see an endocrinologist, your GP may start you on a beta-blocker treatment that damps down overactivity in the nervous system, which can reduce anxiety and sweating as well as reduce the risk of an abnormally fast heart rate.

✔ **Thyroid nodule.** If you have a thyroid nodule, your doctor is likely to refer you to a thyroid specialist clinic for further investigations.

Part I of this book discusses the details of treatment options, and gives information on which options are considered the best according to United Kingdom guidelines. But no matter what you read here (or anywhere else), always discuss your specific situation with your doctor. This book is designed to help you have more productive conversations with your doctor by explaining the pros and cons of each type of treatment and suggesting questions to ask your doctor if a treatment doesn't seem to work for you as an individual. It cannot, however, act as a substitute for your doctor, who knows all the ins-and-outs of your particular case.

In general, if you experience hypothyroidism (low thyroid function), you take a daily pill to replace the thyroid hormone that your body is lacking. Many people take this type of pill for the rest of their lives, but some people are able to stop taking it after a few years if lab tests prove the condition has righted itself. Chapter 5 discusses the treatment of hypothyroidism in more detail.

Three different treatment options exist for someone with hyperthyroidism (an overactive thyroid). You may take an antithyroid drug, receive a radioactive iodine pill to destroy part of your thyroid tissue, or undergo surgery to remove some or all of your thyroid gland. In the United Kingdom, most doctors recommend antithyroid drugs or radioactive iodine for hyperthyroidism. Surgery is now used much less frequently than in the past and is generally performed only when someone can't have one of the other two treatments. Chapter 6 goes into the specifics about each treatment and explains why your doctor may suggest one treatment over the others, depending on your specific situation.

For patients with thyroid cancer, surgery is often required to remove the whole gland. Radioactive iodine is sometimes also used to destroy any thyroid tissue that remains after the surgery. Chapter 8 discusses the treatment of various types of thyroid cancer.

Someone whose thyroid has nodules may need surgery, may not need treatment at all, or may need a type of treatment that falls between those extremes, such as thyroid hormone replacement or radioactive iodine. See Chapters 7 and 9 for all the details about how your doctor may deal with thyroid lumps and bumps.

Understanding the Consequences of Delaying Treatment

As many people with thyroid conditions are undiagnosed, and many die of other causes without ever discovering their thyroid problem, you may wonder whether the diagnosis and treatment of thyroid problems is really necessary.

In some situations, a thyroid condition is so benign or mild that you don't even notice any symptoms. For example, many people with thyroid nodules never have any other problems except for a little lump on their neck. In those mild cases, treatment is often unnecessary.

But for many other people, thyroid conditions are much more serious, having a significant impact on overall health and quality of life. The section 'Realising the Importance of a Healthy Thyroid,' earlier in this chapter, gives you a sense of some possible consequences of delaying treatment. If you have a low functioning thyroid that is left untreated, you may become so overweight, fatigued, and depressed that you have trouble just doing your daily activities. In contrast, with an overactive thyroid, you may experience significant weight loss, heart trouble, and extreme nervousness. And, of course, thyroid cancer is sometimes life-threatening if left untreated, depending on the type of cancer you have. And a thyroid with many nodules can become so enlarged or misshapen that it affects your ability to swallow or breathe properly.

Unless your symptoms are already extreme, only laboratory blood tests can determine whether treatment for your thyroid condition is really necessary, or not. Given how important this little gland is to your health, both physical and mental, most people are well advised to take any treatment their doctor feels is necessary for their wellbeing.

Giving Your Thyroid a Hand: Healthy Lifestyle Choices

So you or a loved one has a thyroid problem – what next? You start taking a prescription, or you undergo another type of treatment, and you wonder what other things you can do to help yourself along towards better health. Did you do something wrong that led to this problem in the first place? What changes can you make to your diet or lifestyle that will lead to a cure, or at least help improve your symptoms?

We wish we could just tell you that if you ate more wonga-wonga beans and got eight hours of sleep each night, your thyroid would return to perfect health. We could stop writing right now if that were the case. Unfortunately, the line between lifestyle choices and thyroid health isn't so straightforward. Your lifestyle definitely plays a role in your thyroid health, but lifestyle does not seem to cause thyroid conditions in the first place. If you are diagnosed with a hyperactive thyroid, for example, you most likely have the condition because you inherited a certain gene, or group of genes, as we discuss in Chapter 17. But if your life is full of stress, if you sleep only five hours a night, and if you drink lots of caffeine to get through the day, you definitely aren't doing your thyroid any favours. Poor lifestyle choices can aggravate the symptoms of your thyroid condition and making some positive changes to your eating, sleeping, and exercise habits means your thyroid definitely benefits.

In Chapter 15, we suggest how improving your diet, reducing your stress, exercising on a regular basis, and keeping a close eye on other aspects of your lifestyle can help to upgrade your thyroid health.

Paying Special Attention: Pregnant Women, Children, and Older People

Although a consensus statement by a group of British thyroid experts states that screening the healthy adult population for thyroid problems is unjustified, some doctors in the United States believe that everyone should have periodic tests to ensure his or her thyroid is working properly, especially after the age of 30 years. Certain groups of people also need to pay special attention to their thyroid function. Pregnant women, children, and the elderly have even more at stake than other folks when it comes to monitoring thyroid function, and Part IV of this book discusses these three groups in more depth.

Pregnancy has a big impact on a woman's thyroid, whether or not she had a thyroid condition prior to the pregnancy. If she does have a known thyroid condition, her doctor monitors it closely during pregnancy because her treatment is likely to need adjustment. And if she doesn't have a thyroid condition, she and her doctor should watch carefully for signs and symptoms of thyroid problems, which can sometimes appear as a result of the physiological changes she's experiencing.

Not only is a healthy thyroid crucial for the mother during pregnancy, but it's essential for the healthy development of her foetus as well. For details about what to watch for during pregnancy and the types of problems a thyroid condition can create for mother and child, see Chapter 18.

Chapter 19 discusses the importance of thyroid screening after the baby is born. Screening is carried out on all newborn infants because a healthy thyroid is essential for proper mental and physical development. If you're a parent of an infant or young child, take a look at Chapter 19 so you understand what the screening is for, what risks are involved for children of parents with thyroid disease, and how to reduce those risks.

The third group that should pay special attention to thyroid health are people aged 65 and over as the symptoms of a thyroid condition so often mirror symptoms of other ailments. If an older person is known to have a heart or blood pressure problem, a doctor may overlook a possible diagnosis of thyroid disease and attribute its symptoms to another condition. To confuse the issue even more, older people often experience symptoms that are the exact opposite of what is expected with certain thyroid conditions. For example, an older person with an underactive thyroid gland may actually lose weight (instead of gaining weight, which is normally expected), especially if he or she is depressed and loses interest in food.

The goal of this book is to help you preserve and defend your thyroid by telling you what you need to know and what to look out for no matter which stage of life you're going through. The more you know about the signs and symptoms of thyroid disease, the earlier you can alert your doctor to when thyroid function tests are a good idea.

Staying Informed

Doctors don't know everything, and general practitioners (GPs) cannot keep fully up-to-date when new discoveries and treatment breakthroughs are popping up all the time. Between writing this book and the time it's printed, for example, researchers will have carried out hundreds more studies and published new findings that might suggest, or prove something different about thyroid diseases and treatments that this book doesn't cover.

You can now stay on top of the latest discoveries thanks to the speed of the Internet. Appendix B gives you a number of useful Web site addresses that can help you stay up-to-date on thyroid health.

Chapter 2

Feeling Fragile: The Emotional Effects of Thyroid Problems

*T*he term *myxoedema madness* is rarely used nowadays, but the expression was popular when first introduced in 1949, and for many years after. Despite its name, myxoedema is not a disease of rabbits (that's myxomatosis) but is an old-fashioned name referring to an underactive thyroid gland or *hypothyroidism*. Myxoedema madness is a form of dementia or psychosis – often with striking delusions – that occurs in some older people with hypothyroidism. Strangely, myxoedema is often triggered shortly after starting thyroid hormone replacement treatment. Sadly, the term myxoedema madness brings with it the suggestion that all people with low thyroid function are somehow mad. Thankfully, that's not the case, and I correct this misconception in this chapter.

As Chapter 3 explains more fully, there's no question that the abnormal production of thyroid hormones can cause changes in someone's mood, and that these changes are sometimes severe. But rarely do you find that someone's mood changes prove so bad they need to go into hospital. Once their over- or underactive thyroid gland is diagnosed and treated, most people suffering from mood problems related to thyroid function respond very well and go on to live perfectly normal lives – both psychologically and physically. Interestingly, however, some people without thyroid problems also benefit from treating their depression with thyroid hormones.

This chapter looks at the current level of understanding about how changes in the production of thyroid hormones (both over- and underproduction) can affect your personality. You discover how often personality or mood disorders are associated with thyroid abnormalities and why thyroid hormones play a role in the treatment of depression, even when no thyroid problem exists.

Because the emphasis in this chapter is on the psychology of thyroid abnormalities, the physical signs and symptoms are not covered; those discussions occur later in the book, primarily in Chapters 5 and 6.

Exploring How an Underactive Thyroid Slows Your Thoughts

Sarah is a 44-year-old woman who is not quite acting as normal, and has not seemed like herself for several months. Her husband, Milton, notices that she is much less talkative than before. She often forgets to pick up the food that they need at the supermarket or to stop at the dry cleaner's to collect clothes that she's dropped off.

Milton wants to discuss a holiday with Sarah, but she doesn't seem to care. Sarah is usually the one responsible for making plans with their friends, but she has not made any for months. Everything she does seems to take more time than it used to, like preparing dinner or getting ready to go to bed. When she finally gets in bed, she is not particularly interested in having sex anymore. The worst thing is that Sarah, usually a happy person, seems sad a lot of the time.

Worried about all these changes, Milton encourages Sarah to see her general practitioner (GP), who examines her and sends her blood for some laboratory tests. On a return visit a few days later, the doctor tells them that Sarah has hypothyroidism. That is, her thyroid gland is not making enough thyroid hormone. He gives her a prescription for replacement thyroid hormone, and about a month later Sarah is well on her way to becoming her old self. Milton is happy because he's once again living with the Sarah he used to know.

Sarah is an excellent example of the changes in personality that can occur when the body is not producing enough thyroid hormone. Depending upon the level of the deficiency, the changes can range from mild to severe and include:

- Decreased talking
- Memory loss

- ✔ General loss of interest

- ✔ Withdrawal from society

- ✔ General slowing of movement

- ✔ Depression, generally mild but sometimes severe

- ✔ Loss of interest in sex

- ✔ An unusually dark sense of humour, in severe cases

Experiencing any of these mental changes on their own does not mean that you definitely have low thyroid function, but they certainly can suggest that you need a test to find out for sure.

If a lack of thyroid hormone is the cause of these symptoms, then taking the right dose of hormone replacement can reverse them. However, if the symptoms don't improve, then you and your doctor need to look elsewhere for the cause. (See Chapter 5 for a thorough discussion of hypothyroidism.)

Seeing How an Overactive Thyroid Can Trigger Anxiety

Sarah's sister, Margaret, who is five years younger, began showing some big personality changes a few years ago. Previously a fairly even-tempered person, she is now easily excited and loses her temper after fairly mild provocation. Her small children never know when their mother is going to yell at them next. She sometimes bursts out in tears but, if asked, cannot give a reason why.

At other times, Margaret is extremely happy, but she can't explain the reason for that either. When she tries to do a task, she often loses interest rapidly and gets distracted. She cannot sit still for very long and is always moving around and fidgeting. Her memory of recent events is poor.

After a few months of absolute chaos in their home, Margaret and her husband, Fred, go to see their GP about her condition. During an examination, the doctor discovers a number of physical findings, including:

- ✔ A rapid pulse

- ✔ A large thyroid gland

- ✔ A fine tremor in Margaret's fingers

The doctor confirms his findings with lab tests (see Chapter 4). Two days later, the doctor tells the concerned pair that Margaret is suffering from *hyperthyroidism* – her body is producing too much thyroid hormone. He refers her to a specialist who begins treatment with medication, and in three weeks, a definite improvement occurs. After six weeks, Margaret is just about back to normal, so she and Fred take the kids to the circus to make up for all the yelling.

Margaret is an excellent example of the psychological changes that can occur when the body produces excessive levels of thyroid hormone. Some of these changes are:

- ✔ Increased excitability
- ✔ An emotional roller coaster of moods
- ✔ Outbursts of anger for no reason
- ✔ Crying spells
- ✔ A tendency to get easily distracted
- ✔ A very short attention span

Years ago, doctors often saw severe, long-standing cases of hyperthyroidism – patients with huge thyroid glands who were visibly shaky and nervous, unable to sit still for more than a few moments. Such acute cases rarely happen nowadays, as increased awareness means that people consult their doctor much sooner, and their condition is usually diagnosed earlier. In isolated cases, however, severe, prolonged hyperthyroidism may result in hallucinations, both in vision and hearing.

Importantly, you need to be aware that when hyperthyroidism affects older people (for example someone in their 80s), the condition may actually look more like hypothyroidism. An older person with hyperthyroidism may feel sad and depressed, apathetic, and withdrawn from society, and the diagnosis is often missed at first. Chapter 20 looks more closely at how thyroid problems can affect people in later life.

The treatments for hyperthyroidism (check out Chapter 6 for more information) are very effective in reversing all the mental and physical symptoms of the condition – particularly in younger people, who are the ones most likely to get the disease.

Fighting Depression

Depression is a common symptom of a lack of thyroid hormone. And conversely, thyroid hormone may help in the treatment of depression, even

Seeing a thyroid specialist

The management of an underactive thyroid gland is usually straightforward and, in the United Kingdom, all GPs are trained to treat this condition. Your doctor may refer you to a specialist for advice on how to manage your condition if:

✔ Your blood tests suggest that you have an underlying disease of the pituitary gland that is failing to kick-start your thyroid

✔ You are pregnant or have recently had a baby

✔ You have a complex medical history

✔ You are under the age of 16 years

However, the management of an overactive thyroid gland is more complex, and guidelines suggest that once your GP diagnoses an overactive thyroid gland, they refer you to an endocrinologist (physician who specialises in treating hormone problems) for expert care. If you have no obvious clinical features (perhaps the diagnosis was made during a routine medical check-up) you don't need any treatment while on the waiting list. However, if you have clinical features of an overactive thyroid gland (which is generally why people with the condition see their doctor in

the first place) your GP may decide to prescribe a treatment to help stabilise your symptoms until specialist advice is available.

If you're not happy with the management of your thyroid condition, you have the right to request a referral to another doctor for a second opinion. However, try to:

✔ **Work with your doctor.** When you consult a doctor, regard him as the expert – your trusted advisor. Unless something feels wrong about the advice you're getting, follow it to the letter. Get behind your treatment and do all you can to make it successful – only then can you get the best possible results.

✔ **Research your condition**. The more you know about your thyroid problem, the easier you find talking to your doctor about it. After all, that's why you're reading this book.

✔ **Join the British Thyroid Foundation (`www.btf-thyroid.org`)**. The Web site has a members' area so that you can see if you have a specialist in your region who can offer help. You can also write to them using the contact details in Appendix B.

when tests indicate that the person has enough thyroid hormone. The following sections explain the role that thyroid hormone plays in depression.

Finding out if your thyroid is causing depression

Depression is a prominent symptom of thyroid disease, especially hypothyroidism. Therefore, when someone is diagnosed with depression, determining whether thyroid disease is the cause can be important.

Although studies show that the majority of depressed people do not have hypothyroidism, the condition is found in a mild form in as many as 20 per cent of depressed people, more often in women than in men. If hypothyroidism is diagnosed, a doctor first determines whether or not the person is already taking an antidepressant drug that could actually cause hypothyroidism as a side effect (see Chapter 10). Two such drugs are lithium and carbamazepine.

If taking an antidepressant is responsible for the hypothyroidism, two options are available. The patient can stop taking the drug, in which case its contribution to the depression disappears, but the patient may still remain depressed for other reasons (mainly the reasons for which they originally needed the antidepressant now causing the antithyroid side effect). Alternatively, the patient can stay on the drug and receive treatment with thyroid hormone if the doctor feels the drug is helping the depression a great deal and no suitable substitute exists.

If you are receiving treatment for depression and have not been tested for thyroid function, ask your doctor whether you need a thyroid check-up.

Using thyroid hormone to treat depression

Many doctors believe that replacement thyroid hormone has a role in the treatment of depression, even when someone is *euthyroid*, which is the posh way of saying that their thyroid function is normal.

Given on its own, thyroid hormone does not seem to reverse depression in someone who doesn't have a thyroid disease. However, when the thyroid hormone triiodothyronine (see Chapter 3) is given together with an antidepressant drug, the effectiveness of the treatment is often improved. This method is especially true when a person is taking a class of drugs called tricyclic antidepressants. The thyroid hormone is particularly effective in turning people who do not respond to the tricyclic antidepressant, into responders. Thyroid hormone treatment also increases the effectiveness of those drugs when they do work.

Interestingly, in cases where the thyroid hormone is used to help treat depression in patients who do not have thyroid disease, when the treatment is stopped after a few weeks or months, the positive effect persists.

TSH, autoantibodies, and depression

Thyroid abnormalities are often associated with other chemical changes in the blood besides too much or too little thyroid hormone. A person with hypothyroidism, for example, may have too much thyroid-stimulating hormone (TSH) or high levels of thyroid autoantibodies, both of which are explained in Chapter 3. Could these other chemical changes promote depression in some patients?

To date, scientists have found no correlation between levels of these other chemical substances and depression. People may sometimes have high autoantibodies while their thyroid function is normal, in which case they don't experience thyroid-related depression. The level of TSH in the blood does not seem to impact depression either.

Current research indicates that the level of the thyroid hormones themselves affect mood, and the levels of these other substances do not.

Chapter 3

Discovering How Your Thyroid Works

*Y*our thyroid is a unique gland whose activity affects every part of your body. The gland makes *hormones* and sends them out into the bloodstream, which carries them to every cell and organ.

Hormones are substances produced by a gland or tissue and transported by the blood to act on a remote organ or tissue, where they produce an effect. These hormones perform many different functions depending upon the particular organ that responds to them.

This chapter shows you how to locate your thyroid. If you have really sensitive fingertips, and your thyroid is slightly on the large side, you might even manage to feel it – in fact, it's often easily findable in normal women. I also cover in this chapter the names of the various hormones that control the thyroid, and those that the thyroid produces itself, before looking at what thyroid hormones do to help your various internal organs work more efficiently.

This chapter also shows you how to recognise when your thyroid is abnormal in size and shape and what happens to your body when thyroid hormones are produced in quantities that are too large or too small.

By reading this whole chapter, you'll know so much about thyroid function that you'll never suffer from undiagnosed *hamburger hyperthyroidism*, a real disease that results from eating cuts of meat that include the thyroid gland of the cow. Eeeugh.

Locating the Thyroid

Have you ever seen one of those wonderful anatomy books where you peel the layers away, starting with the skin, to see all the inner structures of the body? If you do that with the neck, as soon as you peel away the skin you find a bony, V-shaped notch created by the connection of the inside edges of the collar bones. Basically, the main tissue that surrounds the front and sides of the trachea (windpipe) between this V and your Adam's apple is the thyroid gland. The thyroid is shown in Figure 3-1 with some of the more important surrounding structures.

If you want to find your own thyroid (without peeling away your skin), place your index finger at that bony notch below your Adam's apple and push your finger toward the back of your neck. If you then swallow, you may feel something push up against your finger. That is your thyroid gland.

As you can see in Figure 3-1, the thyroid is shaped a bit like a butterfly (or possibly more like upside-down angel's wings). The wings of the butterfly are called the left and right lobes of the thyroid. Connecting the lobes is the isthmus, a narrow strip of tissue between the two larger parts. A third thyroid lobe called the pyramidal lobe, which is another narrow strip of thyroid tissue rising up from the isthmus, is also sometimes visible.

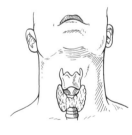

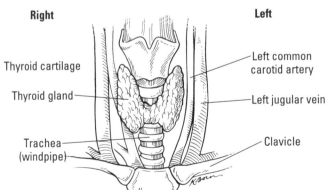

Right   **Left**

Thyroid cartilage

Thyroid gland

Left common
carotid artery

Left jugular vein

Figure 3-1:
The thyroid
gland and
surrounding
anatomy.

Trachea
(windpipe)

Clavicle

When the thyroid is normal in size, it weighs between 10 and 20 grams. That equates to between one-fiftieth and one-twenty-fifth of a pound – not terribly large considering everything it does. Each lobe of the thyroid is only about the size of your thumb. Even so, the thyroid is one of the largest hormone-producing glands in your body.

When looking at the thyroid under a microscope, you can see that it consists of rings of cells one layer deep with a clear centre that acts as a storage depot for the thyroid hormones. These rings are called follicles and are shown in Figure 3-2.

In a developing embryo, the thyroid starts life at the base of the tongue. It then descends to the middle of the neck. In some people, remnants of thyroid still exist at the base of the tongue (known as a lingual thyroid) or along the line of descent.

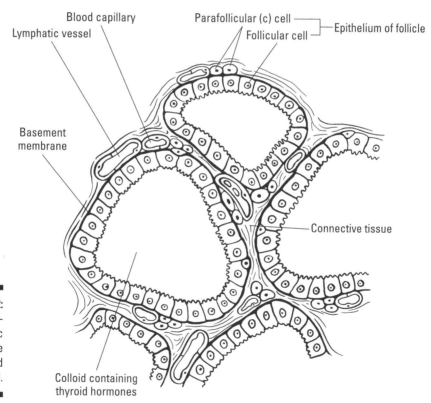

Blood capillary
Lymphatic vessel
Parafollicular (c) cell
Follicular cell
Epithelium of follicle
Basement membrane
Connective tissue
Colloid containing thyroid hormones

Figure 3-2: A microscopic view of the thyroid gland.

Producing Thyroid Hormones

The production of thyroid hormones is regulated by master hormones produced in the brain, as shown in Figure 3-3.

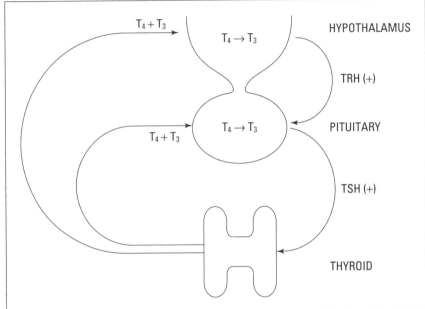

Figure 3-3:
Thyroid
hormone
production.

A part of the brain known as the *hypothalamus* produces a hormone called *thyrotrophin-releasing hormone (TRH)*. This hormone is carried a short distance in the brain to the pituitary gland, where it promotes the release of *thyroid-stimulating hormone (TSH)*.

TSH leaves the pituitary gland and travels in the bloodstream to your thyroid, where it causes the production and release of two thyroid hormones: *thyroxine (T4)* and *triiodothyronine*, which, as they're a bit of a mouthful, are normally known as *T3*. (The numbers 3 and 4 refer to the number of atoms of iodine in the hormones.)

- ✔ T3 is the active form of thyroid hormone.

- ✔ T4 is considered a *prohormone* (literally meaning a 'before hormone'), a much weaker chemical that gains its potency only after being converted to T3.

The conversion of T4 to T3 takes place in many parts of the body (wherever thyroid hormones do their work), not just in the thyroid. The thyroid gland normally releases about 13 times as much T4 as T3. However, overall, you only produce about three times as much T4 as T3. This deficit occurs because most of your T4 is converted into T3 in organs such as the liver, kidneys, and muscles. The thyroid gland itself releases only 20 per cent of the T3 you produce every day.

The statement in the preceding paragraph is profoundly important when treating thyroid hormone deficiencies. Most people with hypothyroidism (low thyroid function) lack both T3 and T4, but during treatment – when taking daily doses of replacement thyroid hormone – they receive only T4. Their bodies must get the T3 they need by converting the T4 into T3. Despite this conversion, these people are still somewhat deficient in T3. Chapter 5 discusses this problem and its possible solutions in more detail in the section 'Taking the right hormones'.

Identifying the importance of iodine

Both T3 and T4 thyroid hormones contain iodine:

- ✔ One molecule of thyroxine (T4) contains four atoms of iodine, which make up 65 per cent of its weight.

- ✔ In contrast, one molecule of triiodothyronine (T3) contains three atoms of iodine, which makes up 58 per cent of its weight.

In fact, your thyroid gland contains the highest concentration of iodine in your body as the gland traps iodine to ensure that it has a ready supply to make its hormones. Because of this fact, the workings of the thyroid are easily studied if radioactive iodine is substituted for regular iodine. In a medical investigation called a *thyroid scan and uptake*, someone with a suspected thyroid problem takes a known dose of radioactive iodine, and the amount that ends up sticking to their thyroid is detected and measured with a refined version of a Geiger counter (see Chapter 4).

Other organs, such as the breasts, the stomach, and the salivary glands, also trap iodine. However, no other organ in your body except the thyroid gland uses iodine for any important purpose, and thyroid hormones are the only significant chemicals you possess that contain iodine.

Regulating thyroid hormones

When thyroid-stimulating hormone (TSH) from your pituitary reaches your thyroid, two things happen:

- ✔ First, the TSH causes the release of existing thyroid hormone into the blood (similar to Blue Peter's famous line of 'Here's one I made earlier').

✔ Second, the TSH prompts the production of more thyroid hormones, both T3 and T4, which collect in the space inside the follicles, awaiting future release. (If your TSH levels are elevated, it can also stimulate overall growth of your thyroid, which can lead to an enlarged thyroid called a goitre.)

The released T3 and T4 circulate throughout your body, reaching, among other places, the pituitary gland. Your pituitary gland has special sensors that detect how much thyroid hormone is present. If the pituitary detects just the right amount, it continues to release the same amount of TSH. If thyroid hormone levels drop for any reason, the pituitary releases more TSH to stimulate the thyroid and tell it to get a move on with making and releasing more thyroid hormone (if it can). However, if the pituitary detects excessive amounts of thyroid hormone, it cuts back on the amount of TSH it produces, so TSH levels fall. This to and fro dialogue between the thyroid and pituitary glands is called the negative feedback for TSH release.

In short, as thyroid hormone falls, TSH rises, and as thyroid hormone rises, TSH falls. Because T3, T4, and TSH are all easily measurable in a blood sample, it's a relatively simple task for laboratory tests to determine the state of your thyroid function (see Chapter 4).

As TSH is also regulated by the release of thyrotrophin-releasing hormone (TRH) from the hypothalamus (see Figure 3-3), the level of TSH in your blood remains very stable throughout life, and abnormal levels usually mean some disease is present.

Moving thyroid hormones around

After T3 and T4 are released from the thyroid, they don't just travel loosely in your blood to their targets – special proteins in the bloodstream carry them. Because 99.97 per cent of thyroid hormone is attached to proteins, only 0.03 per cent floats freely in your circulation.

Only the free thyroid hormone can leave your blood and enter your cells. The rest is solidly bound to proteins and is not available to perform the actions of thyroid hormone – essentially, it's inactive. When a doctor measures the total thyroid hormone in your blood, she measures bound hormone along with the unbound hormone. If she only knows the total T4 amount in your blood, she needs to order a second test to determine the unbound T4 – the hormone that is free in your blood. This second test is important because many drugs and diseases alter the blood levels of thyroxine-binding proteins – the proteins that thyroid hormones bind to. If a drug like oestrogen, for example, increases the amount of thyroxine-binding proteins in your body, your thyroid makes

Proteins that carry thyroid hormones

Three different proteins carry thyroid hormones around your body. The most important by far is thyroxine-binding globulin, responsible for carrying 75 per cent of thyroid hormones in your blood. Transthyretin, previously known as thyroxine-binding prealbumin, carries 20 per cent of your thyroid hormones, while thyroxine-binding albumin carries the other 5 per cent.

Exactly why proteins carry thyroid hormones is not clear. Thyroid hormones that are bound to proteins are inactive and one theory is that having so much tied up with proteins means that an increase in the thyroid gland's hormone output does not result in an increase in thyroid activity. Another theory is that the combination of the hormone and the protein produces a large molecule, which cannot escape from the body through the urine, thus preserving iodine.

more thyroid hormone to bind to these proteins, keeping the unbound thyroid hormone constant and normal. Yet the results of a total T4 blood test will be elevated. Conversely, testosterone, the male hormone, causes a decrease in the thyroxine-binding proteins. If your testosterone level rises, your thyroid makes less thyroxine and a measurement of total T4 shows a decrease (while the unbound T4 again remains normal).

Understanding the Function of Thyroid Hormones

Your thyroid hormones affect just about every cell and organ in your body. They perform general functions that increase the efficiency of each organ's specific functions, whatever they are. This section tells you all about those functions and explains what too much or too little of the thyroid hormones can do to a healthy person.

Many of these changes are caused by other factors besides too little or too much thyroid hormone. For example, an infection can raise your body temperature just as having too much thyroid hormone does. Also, if you have a condition that is associated with dry skin like eczema, or the menopause, this symptom may predominate even if you have hyperthyroidism, which tends to cause moist skin. The information here shows you what classic symptoms of thyroid problems look like, but everyone is different, and each person with the condition may show individual variations.

General functions

Thyroid hormones cause every cell in your body to make more *enzymes*, the proteins that promote your metabolism as they act as the key to help certain chemical reactions take place. If you think of your body as a machine, then adding extra thyroid hormone is like pressing harder on the accelerator of a car. The result is a revving up of the machine – like going from 2,000 revolutions per minute to 4,000 or more revolutions per minute, depending on the amount of hormone added. In the same way, when more thyroid hormone is present in your body, more chemical reactions are taking place.

Metabolism

Your *basal metabolic rate* (BMR) is an overall measure of the amount of chemical reactions taking place in your body. Increased thyroid hormone may increase your BMR, or metabolism, as much as 60 to 100 per cent. Any machine that increases its activity heats up. Likewise, your body heats up when you make more thyroid hormone, and the result is a higher body temperature. At the other end of the scale, not enough thyroid hormone results in an abnormally low body temperature.

As more metabolism takes place, more of your food intake is burned for energy, so less energy is available for storage. Your body detects the need for more energy and you get hungrier, but your faster metabolism usually more than offsets any increase in food intake. The net result is that you lose weight. However, if you take in too much extra food, you can actually gain weight.

 A scientist defines an individual's basal metabolic rate (BMR) as the energy expended when lying in bed, at complete physical and mental rest, 12–14 hours after last eating, in an ambient temperature of 26–30 °C. Although BMR is dependent on thyroid function, metabolism also varies depending on gender (usually higher in males), age (slows as you get older), lean body mass percentage (how much muscle you have), and nutritional status and genetic inheritance (which dictates the efficiency of your metabolism). The type of food you eat also plays a role as heat released during digestion (known as *dietary-induced thermogenesis*) accounts for 10 per cent or more of the energy you get from different foods.

Muscle function

Although your muscles need thyroid hormone for proper functioning, too much of the hormone is not a good thing. Excess thyroid hormone results in muscle wasting, as muscle tissue is consumed as an emergency energy source. As you lose muscle, you become weaker. If too much thyroid hormone is present, the nerves sending signals to your muscles also show increased excitability, resulting in increased reflexes and muscle tremors.

Some unscrupulous diet regimes give unsuspecting people thyroid hormones to speed up their metabolism and help them lose weight. Although this tactic sounds like a good idea, it definitely isn't. An overabundance of thyroid hormone results in muscle loss, so the weight you lose is not fat but muscle, the so-called lean tissue of the body. You do not want to lose lean tissue, as this loss makes you less fit, says goodbye to a toned silhouette, and increases your general flabbiness. Do not use thyroid hormone in an attempt to lose weight.

Energy sources

As well as affecting the protein found in muscle, thyroid hormone also affects the other sources of energy in your body, namely carbohydrates and fats. Carbohydrates are the main source of immediately available energy in the body, so they get used up faster than normal when thyroid hormone levels rise, again resulting in more heat production. Fat is also used up faster than normal. The result is a lowering of the different kinds of fat in the body, namely cholesterol and triglycerides. On the other hand, when thyroid hormone levels drop, the fats accumulate in the liver and the level of cholesterol in the blood rises.

Because chemical reactions require vitamins, minerals, and trace elements, your need for these substances increases when you have more thyroid hormone. Increased thyroid hormones cause a more rapid breakdown of the vitamins. However, multivitamin and minerals supplements have little effect upon the thyroid gland itself, except for those products that contain iodine (often in the form of kelp or seaweed). Supplements and foods containing iodine are best avoided when you have hyperthyroidism or multinodular goitre (see Chapter 9) where extra iodine is used to make too much thyroid hormone.

Specific functions

Every organ in your body requires thyroid hormone to work normally. When that hormone is lacking, the organ tends to carry out less of its usual function, and when too much thyroid hormone is present, the organ does more than it should. In this section, we discuss the most important changes due to abnormal amounts of thyroid hormone in your body. This discussion is not complete by any means, as that needs a large book in itself, and many of the changes that occur are too subtle to result in signs or symptoms that are detectable.

The heart

Your heart needs T4 thyroid hormone for proper pumping. If not enough T4 is present, your heart slows down and its pumping action decreases. This state can even result in heart failure when T4 is severely lacking. Conversely, when T4 levels rise too high, the heart beats too rapidly. While the heart pumps out more blood at first, if this increased pumping continues for too long, it can lead to decreased heart strength so the heart pumps out less blood than normal. This problem occurs because excessive T4 causes muscle wasting, and your heart, of course, is made of muscle.

Depending on your level of physical activity, your normal resting heart rate is usually between 60 and 80 beats per minute (assuming that you're not taking any drugs that affect your pulse). Someone who is in exceptionally good physical condition, such as a trained athlete, may have a heart rate in the 50s or below. People with too much T4, however, often have a heart rate of 120 or faster.

The lungs

As your metabolism increases, you need more oxygen so that the chemical reactions in your body can take place. Oxygen comes into your body through the lungs. Your respiration rate, normally about 16 breaths per minute, has to speed up to bring in more oxygen if you have an overactive thyroid gland. However, even an increased respiration rate may fail to provide you with enough oxygen if your muscular diaphragm and chest muscles are wasting from excess T4.

The stomach and intestines

Your stomach and intestines are linked with muscles that need T4 to push food along for digestion and excretion. When not enough T4 is present, intestinal movement slows, as does the rate at which you absorb nutrients from your food. And slowed bowel movements lead to – yes, you've guessed it – constipation. On the other hand, having too much T4 on board speeds up your bowels, which become looser, more frequent, and can lead to diarrhoea. Great.

The skin, hair, and nails

The increased blood flow that results from a raised level of T4 is especially prominent in the skin. People with hyperthyroidism often have skin that feels warm, they may look flushed, and perspiration may increase, so it also feels moist. When T4 levels fall, the skin is more likely to feel dry and scaly and feels cold to the touch. The nails don't achieve their proper toughness without enough thyroid hormone and may seem brittle with a tendency to break easily. Similarly, the hair is fragile, and excessive hair loss is a common complaint when not enough T4 is present.

The brain and cerebral functioning

Someone with excessive T4 may feel as if her brain is racing, which can result in extreme nervousness. She may feel anxious without knowing why and worry about minor things. In extreme cases, this anxiety can lead to paranoia. In contrast, not enough T4 can lead to mental dullness and depression. Chapter 2 details the changes in mood that can occur with too much or too little thyroid hormone.

Sexual functioning and menstruation

Thyroid hormone is needed for normal sexual function. Both men and women lose interest in sex when not enough T4 is present. They don't necessarily have increased interest in sex when T4 levels rise, however, as so many psychological and physical problems result from the increase.

The menstrual cycle also depends on adequate T4 to proceed normally. Women with a lack of T4 may have trouble conceiving a baby. They tend to have increased menstrual flow and may develop anaemia (from losing too much blood). Too much T4 can also decrease the menstrual flow or cause missed periods.

The bones

Thyroid hormones help bones to grow normally. When too little thyroid hormone is present in early life, the bones show delayed development and do not grow to their correct length. Someone with this condition (dwarfism) is unusually short, with short arms and legs and a larger trunk. If thyroid hormone is lacking after growth has stopped, the bones appear more dense than normal because of decreased bone turnover.

When too much thyroid hormone is present, whether it's due to taking too much thyroid hormone or inadequate treatment of hyperthyroidism, bone turnover and bone loss increases. This disorder can resemble *osteoporosis*, which is the kind of bone loss that occurs in women after the menopause and leads to brittle bones. However, bone thinning associated with excess T4 rarely results in bone fractures once the increased thyroid hormone is controlled with treatment, as the excessive bone loss then stops.

Chapter 4

Testing Your Thyroid

. . . .

In This Chapter

▶ Determining your thyroid hormone levels

▶ Using blood chemicals other than hormones to make a diagnosis

▶ Checking the size, shape, and content of your gland

▶ Investigating abnormal lumps and bumps on the thyroid

. . . .

*T*hese days, taking the precise measurement of thyroid function for granted is easy to do. Yet only 60 years ago, diagnosis depended more upon the physical and emotional state of the person than primitive laboratory tests. As a result, only people with obvious signs and symptoms received a diagnosis – just the tip of a huge iceberg of thyroid abnormalities.

Today, tests that measure thyroid function are getting more and more sensitive. Doctors can identify many people with *subclinical* thyroid disease, meaning their condition is not yet bad enough to trigger symptoms or signs that are apparent to the doctor or patient. These abnormalities are often picked up during routine screening tests and usually progress to become clinical sooner or later. These sensitive tests are therefore invaluable in differentiating problems due to thyroid abnormalities with the symptoms of ageing (such as general slowing down), which are so similar to those of mild hypothyroidism.

As thyroid disorders are so common, laboratories receive around 10 million requests for thyroid function tests per year in the United Kingdom, costing an estimated £30 million! Although you cannot order these tests for yourself (you request them through your doctor), this information can increase your understanding of what various tests involve and what their results mean. The material covered in this chapter can also help you have better discussions with your doctor about your diagnosis.

Checking Blood Levels of Thyroid Hormones

Numerous blood tests are available to measure thyroid function, but the most accurate and sensitive tests for determining thyroid function are the *free thyroxine* (FT4) and the *thyroid-stimulating hormone* (TSH) tests, both of which are described in this section. (Free thyroxine is the tiny portion of thyroid hormone in the blood that is not bound to protein and is therefore free to enter your cells; refer to Chapter 3.) The vast majority of people are accurately diagnosed with these tests. If you're undergoing screening for thyroid function and your doctor wants to order just one test to start, that test is usually the TSH due to its accuracy and the fact that it's a simple blood test.

Many doctors practising today learned about thyroid disease years ago, when only older tests were available, and they still use them. Just in case your doctor orders such tests or in case you have copies of old test results that you want to understand, this section also explains how some of the older tests work.

Total thyroxine

The *total thyroxine* or *TT4* test (sometimes called the *T4 immunoassay*) measures all the T4 thyroid hormone in a given quantity of blood. But, most of the hormone measured (more than 99 per cent) is inactive because it is bound to protein (refer to Chapter 3). So, by itself, this test does not tell you how much thyroid activity is present. This test can only give a more accurate picture of active thyroid hormone function if the test is combined with a test that measures what per cent of the total thyroxine is bound and what per cent is free.

Seeing what raises TT4

The total thyroxine test is also deceiving at times. Many drugs and clinical states raise the level of TT4 in your blood, by raising the amount of thyroxine-binding protein present, although they don't impact the amount of free thyroxine. Some of the drugs that can raise the level of TT4 in your blood include:

- **Oestrogen hormones:** Used in hormone replacement therapy (HRT) and the oral contraceptive pill
- **Amiodarone:** A drug used for the heart
- **Amphetamines:** Stimulant drugs
- **Methadone:** An opiate drug
- **Phenothiazines:** A class of drugs used to treat some psychiatric conditions, such as schizophrenia

Some clinical states that raise TT4 levels include:

- ✔ High oestrogen states, such as pregnancy
- ✔ Acute illness, such as AIDS or hepatitis
- ✔ Acute psychiatric problems

Understanding what lowers TT4

Conversely, some drugs and physical conditions tend to lower the results of a TT4 test by reducing the amount of thyroxine-binding protein you make, without affecting the amount of free thyroxine in your circulation. The drugs that have this impact include:

- ✔ **Androgens:** Male hormones taken to build muscle
- ✔ **Corticosteroids:** Usually given to reduce inflammation
- ✔ **Nicotinic acid:** Given to lower harmful blood fats

Physical conditions that can lower TT4 levels include:

- ✔ Severe chronic illness, such as kidney failure or liver failure
- ✔ Starvation or severe malnutrition

Some medicines, such as non-steroidal anti-inflammatory drugs (NSAIDs), phenytoin (used to treat epilepsy), and aspirin, can also displace thyroid hormones from their binding proteins to reduce the total but not the free thyroid hormone concentrations, once a new steady state is reached. So, if thyroid status is tested in someone taking one of these drugs who isn't in a steady state with their treatment (perhaps because they recently started therapy or the dose was recently changed) the results are misleading.

Looking at what's normal for TT4

The normal range of TT4 is usually around 60–160 nmol/L (nanomoles per litre) of blood.

Different laboratories may use different techniques to perform the same test, resulting in slightly different normal values. Even when they use the same technique, slight variations in the normal values often appear from lab to lab. Each lab uses its own reference group of people without thyroid disease who act as guinea pigs for the lab to draw up their normal range. Most test result sheets include the laboratory's reference range next to the person's own individual blood test result, which makes interpreting what's happening easier. With the availability of reliable tests for free T4, the justification for laboratories to continue using the TT4 test is diminishing.

How the resin T3 uptake is done

When radioactive T3 or T4 is mixed with your blood in a test tube, it combines with the binding sites on the thyroxine-binding proteins. Your blood is then exposed to a substance called a resin that binds the unbound T3 or T4, and the resin is measured for radioactivity. The result is expressed as the per cent of radioactivity found on the resin, compared to the original radioactivity that was added. The more binding sites available on your proteins, the lower the resin uptake result, and vice versa.

If your doctor chooses to use the total thyroxine test to monitor your thyroid function, however, he first makes certain that you aren't taking any of the drugs or experiencing any of the physical conditions listed in this section. In addition, your doctor must also order the next test, the resin T3 uptake, to get a complete picture of how much of the total T4 measured is tied up to protein, and how much remains free and active in your circulation.

Resin T3 uptake

The *resin T3 uptake* test is now virtually obsolete. This test measures whether your thyroxine-binding proteins have a lot of spare sites for T3 hormone (active thyroid hormone) to bind on to. This occurs when the TT4 is low (and therefore taking up very few of the sites) or when the binding protein levels are very high.

The effect of any of the drugs or physical conditions that reduce the binding sites (flip back to the section 'Understanding what lowers TT4') – thus, causing a low TT4 measurement – leaves very few binding sites for any more thyroid hormone to bind to. If T3 is added to a sample of that blood, little T3 can bind, leaving a lot of measurable free T3. The resin T3 uptake is therefore high. Any of the drugs or clinical states that raise the binding sites (refer back to the section 'Seeing what raises TT4') – thus, causing an increased TT4 level – also leaves a lot of binding sites available for added T3. The amount of free T3 measured is then low, giving a decreased resin T3 uptake. The usual result of a resin T3 uptake is 25–35 per cent depending on the laboratory.

Free thyroxine index

As the previous sections discuss, the total thyroxine (TT4) test and the resin T3 uptake are used together for greatest value, as several drugs and physical conditions can alter the results of the TT4 test (and also alter the resin T3 uptake results). The impact of such drugs and physical conditions always affects the TT4 and resin T3 uptake results in opposite directions: If the TT4 is depressed, then the resin T3 uptake is high; if the TT4 is elevated, the resin T3 uptake is low.

To help wrap these findings up in one useful result, doctors multiply the TT4 level by the resin T3 uptake. The result is called the *free thyroxine index (FT₄I)* and, depending on the laboratory, the normal range is around 20–63 on the index. A result below the usual reference range for a laboratory indicates low thyroid function, while a result above the usual reference range indicates increased thyroid function.

Even when you are taking one of the drugs or experiencing one of the physical conditions listed in the 'Total thyroxine' section, the free thyroxine index is within the normal range if your thyroid is functioning normally.

Free thyroxine (FT4)

The *free thyroxine* (FT4 or sometimes fT4) test is the best way to measure the amount of free thyroid hormone in your blood. This test measures the 0.03 per cent of T4 that is not bound to protein – the T4 that is free to interact with your cells (refer to Chapter 2). All the factors that can change the amount of total thyroxine in your system, such as the drugs and physical conditions listed earlier in this chapter, do not affect the amount of FT4 in your blood. Depending upon the test method that is used by the particular laboratory, the usual FT4 level is around 9.0 to 25 pmol/L (picomols per litre).

The level of FT4 in your blood is high if you have hyperthyroidism and low if you have hypothyroidism. (As Chapter 6 explains in more detail, in rare cases, a person with hyperthyroidism has too much T3 rather than too much T4 in his blood. In these rare instances, an FT4 test could come back normal or even low.)

The FT4 is not a perfect test, because certain conditions do arise that make the FT4 level appear abnormal when the patient actually has normal thyroid function. Fortunately, these conditions are easily recognised. They include the following:

- Having severe chronic illness (not thyroid disease), such as kidney or liver failure, may slightly decrease FT4.

- Producing or ingesting large amounts of T3 – through excessive thyroid medication, for example – decreases FT4.

- Having a rare condition, often hereditary such as one of the rare inherited conditions discussed in Chapter 17, in which there is a resistance to T4, causing high levels of FT4 in someone who is not yet hyperthyroid.

- Receiving the drug heparin to prevent blood clotting may slightly increase FT4.

- Having an acute illness, such as AIDS or hepatitis, may briefly elevate FT4 as binding proteins suddenly fall.

Free triiodothyronine (FT3)

The *free triiodothyronine (FT3)* test measures the free T3 hormone in the blood. This test is rarely necessary, except in the situation where a person is obviously hyperthyroid, yet their FT4 test result is normal. The usual level of FT3 is 3.5 to 7.7 pmol/L (picomols per litre). Someone with hyperthyroidism has a high FT3 result, while a person with hypothyroidism has a low FT3 value.

Thyroid-stimulating hormone (TSH)

In most circumstances, the *thyroid-stimulating hormone (TSH)* test is the most sensitive test of thyroid function. The body's own negative feedback system means that TSH rises when the T4 level in the blood falls, and the TSH falls when the T4 rises (refer to Chapter 3). The assays that measure TSH are among the most accurate clinical techniques currently available, making them a reliable test to measure thyroid function. If you have hyperthyroidism, your TSH level is low (because TSH production is suppressed by the high level of T4 in your blood). If you have hypothyroidism, your TSH level is high (because your body is trying to stimulate production of more T4).

Seeing what lowers TSH levels

Many different conditions can cause a reduction in your TSH level, and having a low TSH does not necessarily mean that you have hyperthyroidism. The factors that can decrease your TSH include:

- ✔ Receiving excessive treatment with T3 or T4 hormone

- ✔ Developing thyroid nodules, which make excessive T3 or T4 (see Chapter 6)

- ✔ During the first three months of pregnancy. (A hormone called *human chorionic gonadotrophin* is produced during this time, which has TSH-like properties and stimulates the production of T4, thereby suppressing TSH.)

- ✔ Suffering from the cancers known as *choriocarcinoma* or molar pregnancy, both of which are associated with the production of large amounts of the hormone, human chorionic gonadotrophin

- ✔ Having a pituitary tumour that destroys TSH producing cells

- ✔ Developing Euthyroid (normal thyroid function) Graves' disease, where hyperthyroidism is present in the thyroid but the thyroid is not making levels of T4 that are excessive (see Chapter 5)

- ✔ Suffering from acute depression

Understanding what raises TSH levels

Several conditions can cause an increase in your TSH level, even if your thyroid is not underactive. The following conditions have to be considered when a high TSH is found:

- ✔ Presence of a pituitary tumour involving the cells that make TSH
- ✔ Recovery from a severe illness
- ✔ Insufficient dietary iodine
- ✔ Resistance to the action of T4
- ✔ Failure of the adrenal gland to make adrenal hormone
- ✔ Psychiatric illness

Looking at what's normal for TSH

Depending on the particular laboratory doing the test, a normal TSH level is 0.3–4.5 µU/ml (microunits per millilitre).

Many of the conditions listed in this section are temporary, meaning that a person's TSH levels return to normal in time. Other conditions, such as a pituitary tumour, require action (in this case, the removal of the tumour) to restore the TSH to its normal level.

Sometimes, a condition that suppresses production of TSH, such as hyperthyroidism, produces a low TSH level for a period of time even after you've returned to a normal metabolic state with treatment. The FT4 is normal, but the TSH remains low. This instance is one occasion when the TSH is not a reliable guide to thyroid function, so the FT4 is used instead.

After your doctor establishes a diagnosis for a thyroid problem, you may have repeated TSH tests during the course of your treatment to monitor your progress. If you are having treatment for hyperthyroidism, however, repeated TSH tests are not always the most effective way to monitor progress, because your TSH may not recover for a long time after your metabolism returns to normal.

Taking Non-Hormonal Blood Tests

Having thyroid disease does not necessarily mean that your thyroid is over- or underactive. For example, a person with thyroid inflammation or thyroid cancer could have normal levels of FT4 and TSH even though they have a thyroid problem. In this situation, blood tests other than those described in the previous section are helpful in making the correct diagnosis. This section helps you understand when these tests are necessary and how you interpret their results.

Thyroid autoantibodies

Many thyroid conditions fall into the category of *autoimmune thyroid diseases* – such as autoimmune thyroiditis (also known as chronic thyroiditis or Hashimoto's thyroiditis (see Chapter 5)), and Graves' disease (see Chapter 6) – as they appear to result from the body rejecting its own tissue. Under a microscope, diseased thyroid tissue contains many of the same immune cells that are found when a foreign invader is present in the body, for example when an organ is transplanted from one person to another.

The tissue, cell, or chemical that the body is trying to reject is known as an *antigen*. One of the types of special proteins that the body manufactures to reject an antigen is called an *antibody*. When an antibody is directed against your own tissue, it is called an *autoantibody* (an antibody directed against yourself).

When you have an autoimmune thyroid disease, many autoantibodies are found in your body, but the two principal ones are called *antithyroglobulin autoantibody* and *antimicrosomal* (now called *thyroid peroxidase*) *autoantibody*. Antiperoxidase autoantibodies are found more often than antithyroglobulin autoantibodies. One other autoantibody is also important in people who have hyperthyroidism. This autoantibody is the thyroid-stimulating immunoglobulin (TSI) that acts like TSH in stimulating the thyroid to make and release more hormones.

If your doctor wants to confirm a diagnosis of an autoimmune thyroid disease, he orders tests to look for antithyroid autoantibodies and thyroid peroxidase autoantibodies. If either test returns at a level of over 100 international units per millilitre, the diagnosis is confirmed.

These autoantibodies are found at the highest levels in people with a condition called *Hashimoto's thyroiditis* (which Chapter 5 explains in more detail), but they are also found in people with *Graves' disease*, a form of hyperthyroidism (see Chapter 6). Interestingly, thyroid autoantibodies are found at lower levels in up to 10 per cent of normal people (the percentage increases with age). Some thyroid specialists even believe that people with low levels of autoantibodies actually have subclinical (non-symptomatic) thyroid disease. If this belief is true, the population with thyroid disease is far greater than previously thought.

If autoantibodies are not present in abnormal amounts, a diagnosis of Hashimoto's thyroiditis is not appropriate.

Although each autoimmune disease of the thyroid is discussed in its own chapter in this book, the diseases are really just different clinical presentations of the same underlying condition. The evidence for this statement is based on the following facts:

- ✔ The thyroid tissue appears the same in the different conditions.

- ✔ Autoimmune thyroid disease runs in families.

- ✔ One person may pass through Graves' disease, Hashimoto's disease, and hypothyroidism at different times.

- ✔ The same types of autoantibodies are found in all three groups.

Some autoantibodies stimulate the thyroid, while others suppress the thyroid. At any given time, the condition of someone with an autoimmune disease of the thyroid depends upon which group of antibodies is present at the highest levels. When more suppression than stimulation is present, the person has low thyroid function. When more stimulation than suppression is present, the person has hyperthyroidism. Someone may start with an overactive thyroid gland due to excess stimulation by autoantibodies, go back to normal, and then end up with low thyroid function due to over suppression. Treatment sometimes does nothing more than speed up this process.

Finding autoantibodies is a clue that thyroid disease is likely in the future. Relatives of people with an autoimmune thyroid disease often have autoantibodies themselves, and many of them go on to develop thyroid disease at some point in their life.

In up to 25 per cent of people with an autoimmune thyroid disease, the condition goes away after a time. A higher concentration of autoantibodies does not mean that a patient is sicker than someone who has a lower concentration. This state may simply mean that the illness is less likely to go away.

Serum thyroglobulin

Thyroglobulin is the form in which thyroid hormones are packaged within the thyroid, and this complex of hormone bound to protein occupies most of the centre of each thyroid follicle (refer to Chapter 3). Thyroglobulin is broken down to release thyroid hormones when more is needed. Thyroglobulin is found in the blood of normal individuals, but its level is much higher when thyroid damage is present (for example, with cancer of the thyroid or inflammation of the thyroid). A normal level of thyroglobulin varies from laboratory to laboratory but is typically between 3 and 42 µg/L (micrograms per litre).

Doctors don't test the level of thyroglobulin in your blood for the purpose of making a diagnosis, because several different conditions cause elevations. Rather, this test is used to follow the course of a person already diagnosed

Theories explaining autoantibody production

Exactly why the body forms antibodies against its own tissue is not known, but several theories exist. Ordinarily, cells in the body are present to prevent production of antibodies against the self. One suggestion is that people who form thyroid autoantibodies are deficient in those protective cells at some point early in life.

Another suggestion is that a foreign invader (like a virus) may have antigens similar to those found in thyroid tissue. In making antibodies to fight this foreign invader, and its foreign antigens, the body may accidentally make antibodies that fight its own tissue as well.

with a thyroid condition – especially someone with thyroid cancer, who shows an increase in thyroglobulin if their cancer grows and spreads. Immediately after surgery for thyroid cancer, the thyroglobulin level is very low, but if the cancer remains present and spreads, the thyroglobulin increases, providing a useful monitoring tool.

Determining the Size, Shape, and Content of Your Thyroid

As discussed earlier in this chapter, levels of free thyroxine (FT4) and thyroid-stimulating hormone (TSH) are normal in people who have thyroid conditions where hormone activity is normal. Therefore, other types of test are necessary to gather information about the size, shape, and content of your thyroid gland. And, when your doctor diagnoses abnormal thyroid activity, one or more of these studies may help to identify the underlying cause. Each test is easy and painless and provides information that is unobtainable in any other way.

Radioactive iodine uptake and scan

Your thyroid concentrates iodine from your blood in order to make thyroid hormones, scooping up so much that it boasts the richest concentration of iodine in your body (refer to Chapter 3). This concentration makes a ready target for studying the dynamic activity of this important gland.

If someone receives *radioactive iodine* (in the form of a capsule to swallow) and a device such as a Geiger counter is passed over the thyroid gland that device can accurately count the level of radioactivity present. These counts of radioactivity are registered on paper as dots, giving the radiologist a useful join-the-dots puzzle for his coffee break. A normal thyroid appears like a butterfly at the lower end of the neck (refer to Chapter 3). If the gland is functioning normally, dots in every part of the gland are uniform and the picture on paper shows the shape and two-dimensional size of the gland.

If a single thyroid nodule is present, and is overactive, most of the radioactive iodine concentrates in that nodule, giving it a darker appearance on paper. Because of this appearance, that spot of the thyroid is called a *hot nodule*. The rest of the gland is often suppressed and appears lighter; therefore it's said to be 'cold'. If the nodule itself does not concentrate as much iodine as the rest of the gland, it's called a *cold nodule*. Thyroid cancers are generally 'cold', because cancerous parts of the thyroid do not produce thyroid hormone in the usual way. However, most cold nodules are not cancer.

In addition to showing the size and shape of the gland, a radioactive scan and uptake measures the relative activity of the thyroid. When the thyroid is overactive, it takes up more iodine than normal. When the thyroid is underactive, it takes up less than normal. The maximum uptake of radioactivity usually occurs about 24 hours after swallowing the iodine. At this point, a normal thyroid has taken up between 5 and 25 per cent of the administered dose of iodine. An overactive thyroid takes up 35 per cent or more. An uptake between 25 and 35 per cent is a borderline reading.

Figure 4-1 shows the appearance of a normal thyroid scan and a scan that indicates hyperthyroidism. The second scan is much darker and shows a larger thyroid gland, consistent with the increased uptake and growth of the thyroid in hyperthyroidism.

Figure 4-1:
A normal thyroid and a hyperactive thyroid as shown in a radioactive iodine scan.

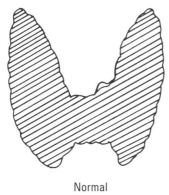

Normal

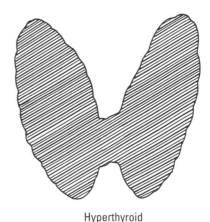

Hyperthyroid

A few situations can arise that affect the results of a thyroid scan and uptake. Someone taking large amounts of iodine – for example if taking a drug which contains iodine, such as amiodarone – causes both the iodine uptake within the thyroid to be blocked and dilutes the administered dose. Taking thyroid replacement hormone also blocks thyroid activity and reduces the uptake of radioactive iodine. Diseases, such as silent thyroiditis (see Chapter 12) where the iodine leaves the thyroid rapidly, also prevent a proper study.

The radioactive iodine scan and uptake generally used to be carried out to diagnose an overactive thyroid. The test is now uncommon as the blood levels of T4 and TSH are usually definitive and, along with the physical examination, are enough to confirm the diagnosis. The scan and uptake is now used more often to establish whether a thyroid that's abnormal in shape contains multiple nodules (see Chapter 9) and to determine whether any of those nodules is overactive.

Rather than swallowing radioactive iodine by mouth, an alternative is to receive an injection of radioactive technetium, directly into a vein, 30 minutes before the scan.

Thyroid ultrasound

The *thyroid ultrasound*, also known as an *echogram* or *sonogram*, is a study that uses sound to measure the size, shape, and consistency of thyroid tissue. No radiation is used in an ultrasound study.

During this test, you lie on your back on a table with your neck hyperextended (chin right up in the air as far as you can). A gel is placed on the neck to help the transmission of sound waves. A device called a *transducer* is then passed over the area of the thyroid, sending out high-pitched sound waves that are reflected back by your tissues and collected via a microphone. Tissue that contains water gives the best reflections, while solid tissue like bone gives poor reflections.

A thyroid ultrasound can measure the size of your thyroid and any nodules very precisely. This test is used to follow treatment for an enlarged thyroid or nodule to see whether it's shrinking. The ultrasound can also tell the difference between a cyst that is filled with fluid (and is almost never a cancer) and a solid nodule, which is sometimes a cancer.

This test is often used after a radioactive iodine scan detects an area that is cold. Is the area cold because it contains no thyroid tissue (which is how a cyst appears), or is the area cold because it contains cancerous thyroid tissue that is solid? The ultrasound can differentiate a cyst from a solid mass but cannot tell you whether the mass is cancer. (Most of the time, cancer is not present.)

Figure 4-2 shows a normal ultrasound study of the thyroid and one with a prominent nodule that is solid.

Normal ultrasound

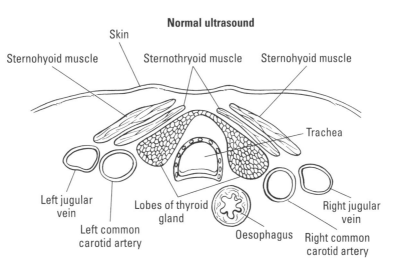

Skin

Sternohyoid muscle

Sternothryoid muscle

Sternohyoid muscle

Trachea

Left jugular vein

Lobes of thyroid gland

Right jugular vein

Left common carotid artery

Oesophagus

Right common carotid artery

Nodule shown on ultrasound

Figure 4-2:
A normal ultrasound study (top) and an ultrasound that shows a solid nodule (bottom).

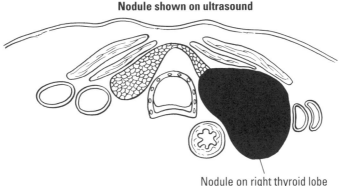

Nodule on right thyroid lobe

Fine needle aspiration biopsy (FNAB)

When a doctor wants to know the type of tissue making up a growth on the thyroid, the *fine needle aspiration biopsy (FNAB)* is the definitive test. This test is virtually painless and is free of complications. A small needle is introduced into the growth, and tiny bits of tissue are sucked up (aspirated) by pulling back on the plunger to create a vacuum. The needle is moved to a few different places on the growth.

The aspirated tissue is sprayed on a fixative, stained, and examined for signs of cancer. This test is a fairly reliable method to establish whether the growth is cancerous or not. Occasionally, the tissue won't provide a clear diagnosis, and the lobe (side) of the thyroid (refer to Chapter 3) that contains the lump is removed in an operation called, simply, a *lumpectomy*.

FNAB has saved thousands of patients from surgery and is often the first test performed to check for cancer, skipping the thyroid scan and the ultrasound. This approach is based on the Willie Sutton theory. Willie was a bank robber and was once asked why he robbed banks. His answer was 'You go where the money is.'

Deciphering ultrasound

A beam of sound from an ultrasound device consists of high frequency sound waves. The frequency is far higher than anything the human ear can hear. When focused and directed, just like a beam of light, to strike tissue, the tissue reflects a certain amount of the sound beam back – the amount depends upon the density of the tissue. Air hardly reflects back any of the beam, while tissue, which is made up of many layers and contains water, sends plenty of sound back. Different tissues absorb the sound differently; therefore, reflecting the sound to a different extent. A cancer appears differently on an ultrasound to a normal thyroid tissue or a cyst filled with fluid. When the reflection returns, the sound energy is converted to light energy and electrical energy. These signals are then displayed on a cathode ray tube or, if a film is exposed to the light energy, made into a permanent record.

Part II
Treating Thyroid Problems

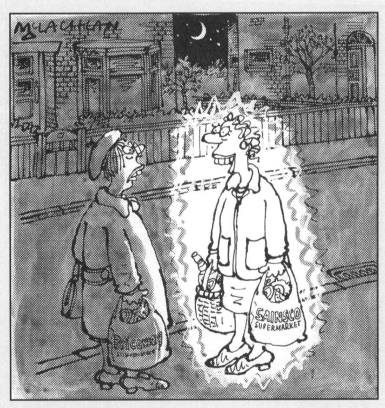

"Now I'm getting better, they're taking me off the radioactive iodine treatment."

In this part . . .

The thyroid can be overactive or underactive. It can be too large or too small. It can be bumpy or smooth. The chapters in this part introduce you to all kinds of thyroid abnormalities. You discover how to recognize them and how to differentiate one from another. For those of you with thyroid disorders, we explain how they occur, which of the common signs and symptoms you have, how a particular disorder damages your body, and what you can do to cure it so no damage occurs.

Chapter 5

Dealing with an Underactive Thyroid

Low thyroid function (also known as hypothyroidism or myxoedema) is the most common form of thyroid disease throughout the world. Although the condition has numerous causes, iodine deficiency leads the list worldwide (see Chapter 12). In the United Kingdom and other parts of Europe, however, iodine deficiency is rare. The leading cause of hypothyroidism is the presence of an autoimmune thyroid disease. An autoimmune condition is one in which your own immune system attacks a part of the body, usually by producing antibodies that recognise and attack a body component such as the thyroid. Autoimmune thyroid conditions include *chronic thyroiditis,* known also as *Hashimoto's thyroiditis* or *autoimmune thyroiditis,* which is discussed in this chapter, and Graves' disease (see Chapter 6). (Check out Chapter 4 for a description of thyroid autoantibodies.)

This chapter introduces you to the immensity of this problem, shows you how hypothyroidism affects the body, and explains the proper treatment for the various forms of hypothyroidism. In the last few years, key changes in our understanding of hypothyroidism have occurred, and that new information is included here, too, so you are up-to-date when you talk with your doctor about symptoms and treatment.

Living with Autoimmune Thyroiditis

Stacy, a 46-year-old woman, is the cousin of Sarah and Margaret, who are introduced in Chapter 2. Stacy is generally healthy but recently noticed some swelling in the lower part of her neck. The swelling seemed to develop very slowly, and she didn't notice it until she tried to button a collar over her neck. Other than the swelling, she has really not had any physical problems. Stacy isn't gaining weight. She sleeps well at night and isn't overly tired. She doesn't feel unusually hot or cold. Her appetite is normal, as are her bowel movements. She has no discomfort associated with the growth in her neck.

Stacy's cousin, Sarah, who was recently diagnosed with hypothyroidism, tells Stacy that, according to her thyroid specialist, other members of her family may develop thyroid disease, too. Stacy goes to see her GP, who examines her and finds that her thyroid gland is twice as large as normal. She finds no other significant abnormalities. She sends Stacy to the nurse for two blood tests – a thyroid-stimulating hormone (TSH) test and a free thyroxine (FT4) test – both of which return within the normal range (refer to Chapter 4). Because of her clinical suspicion, Stacy's GP also obtains thyroid autoantibody studies. These results are very elevated, particularly the thyroid peroxidase autoantibodies, but also the antithyroglobulin autoantibodies (discussed in Chapter 4).

Stacy's doctor tells her that she has a condition called *chronic thyroiditis*. He tells Stacy that treatment at this time is optional. If she is unhappy with the swelling sticking out on her neck, she can take thyroid hormone and it will shrink. If not, she need only return in six months or a year to check whether the disease has progressed to hypothyroidism.

Stacy's condition is a typical illustration of chronic thyroiditis. She is free of symptoms at this stage, and the only abnormality is her goitre, an enlargement of the thyroid gland. The blood tests that reflect thyroid function are normal. The high levels of thyroid autoantibodies in her system determine the diagnosis.

The extent of the problem

Most studies indicate that 10 per cent of the world's population tests positive for thyroid autoantibodies (refer to Chapter 4). If the United Kingdom has a population of approximately 60 million people, around 6 million of them will test positive. Many experts believe that all these people have chronic thyroiditis, but the vast majority will never develop symptoms and the condition won't bother them in any way.

Only about 1 in 1,000 of people who test positive for thyroid autoantibodies develop symptomatic chronic thyroiditis, which means that about 6,000 new cases occur in the United Kingdom each year. A woman is 20 times more liable to develop *symptomatic* chronic thyroiditis – chronic thyroiditis where the symptoms actually show – than a man. The typical patient is 30 to 50 years old, but chronic thyroiditis is also found in children.

Chronic thyroiditis is a familial disease that is usually transmitted from mother to daughter. Even members of the family who show no symptoms often have thyroid autoantibodies in their blood (especially the females). They may develop hypothyroidism later on.

Symptoms of chronic thyroiditis

Some people with chronic thyroiditis do have symptoms, even when their thyroid function tests are normal. In addition to neck swelling, symptoms include:

- Pain in the neck (which is unusual)
- Chest pain (which occurs in about 25 per cent of patients)
- Sensation of fullness in the neck and sometimes, trouble swallowing
- Transient symptoms of hyperthyroidism (see Chapter 6) – but blood tests are not normal when these short-term symptoms occur

Approach to treatment

As the condition is so benign, chronic thyroiditis that has not progressed to hypothyroidism is usually not treated. If you have neck pain because of chronic thyroiditis, it's generally controlled with aspirin or paracetamol. If the swelling in your neck is unsightly, or you have difficulty swallowing, your doctor can prescribe thyroid hormone to block the production of thyroid-stimulating hormone (TSH). Your thyroid gland then shrinks. Your doctor may suggest stopping hormone treatment at some later date, and review you regularly, as one-quarter of patients with this condition have a remission and no longer need thyroid treatment.

If you experience transient symptoms of hyperthyroidism as a result of chronic thyroiditis, these symptoms usually require no treatment either. The symptoms usually last a few weeks, and then you return to normal. In especially severe cases, drugs that block the action of thyroid hormones (see Chapter 6) are used.

Identifying Hypothyroidism

Karen is Stacy's younger sister. Over the last few years, she has noticed a gradual enlargement of her neck – a symptom similar to the one that Stacy experienced. But Karen has had a number of other problems as well. She has gained a few pounds, and her legs appear swollen but do not retain an indentation when she presses on them. She feels cold when her husband feels comfortable and is constantly asking for more heat. Her skin is dry and her nails are brittle. She has dry hair and notices that she is losing more hair than before. The outer third of her eyebrows seems to have disappeared, along with some of her eyelashes. She used to love to sing in the church choir, but her voice is now too husky. She has trouble seeing to drive at night and notices trouble hearing as well.

Her GP, who is familiar with the family's thyroid problems, examines her in her surgery. She finds that, in addition to all the symptoms Karen explains to him, she also has a slow pulse and an enlarged thyroid gland. She sends her for thyroid function tests (TSH and FT4) as well as thyroid autoantibody tests.

Karen's tests show that she has a low FT4, a high TSH and her autoantibody levels are elevated. The doctor makes a diagnosis of hypothyroidism due to chronic thyroiditis and starts her on thyroid hormone replacement. Within six weeks, Karen is back to her old self.

Signs and symptoms of hypothyroidism

Karen illustrates the classic signs and symptoms of hypothyroidism. The signs, including some that Karen did not show, are:

- Slow pulse and enlarged heart
- Enlarged thyroid (goitre), unless prior removal of the thyroid gland is the cause of hypothyroidism
- Dry, cool skin that is puffy, pale, and yellowish
- White patches of skin where pigment is lost (a condition called vitiligo)
- Brittle nails
- Dry, brittle hair that tends to fall out excessively – especially loss of the outer third of the eyebrows
- Swelling that does not retain an indentation, especially of the legs (this condition is known as brawny oedema)
- Hoarseness and slow speech with a thickened tongue
- Expressionless face
- Slow reflexes

People with hypothyroidism complain of many different symptoms, and each person has unique complaints. Among the most common are:

✔ Intolerance to cold

✔ Tiredness and a need to sleep

✔ Weakness

✔ Pain and stiffness in the joints and muscles

✔ Constipation

✔ Increased menstrual flow

✔ Trouble hearing and a ringing in the ears

✔ Trouble seeing at night

The physician who sees someone with these signs and symptoms obtains several tests to confirm the diagnosis. The two test results essential to the diagnosis are:

✔ A free thyroxine (FT4) level that is lower than normal

✔ A thyroid-stimulating hormone (TSH) level that is higher than normal

Other tests that support the diagnosis include:

✔ A mild anaemia (decrease in red blood cells)

✔ An increased cholesterol count

✔ Elevated levels of thyroid autoantibodies (if the patient has autoimmune hypothyroidism)

✔ A blood glucose level that is lower than normal

After the diagnosis of hypothyroidism is made, the various causes of this condition are checked out, as many of them are reversible without treating the thyroid directly.

Confusing conditions

The signs and symptoms of hypothyroidism are fairly non-specific and are easily confused with the signs and symptoms of other common conditions. The three major sources of confusion are menopause, normal ageing, and stress. All three are common occurrences for women, and men experience at least two out of the three (although some doctors also believe that the male menopause exists). You can see how a person with low thyroid function could easily neglect to check for that condition. This fact is a major reason why some doctors suggest routine thyroid testing starting at age 35 and continuing every five years thereafter, although this view is highly controversial as thyroid screening costs a lot of money.

Pinpointing the Causes of Hypothyroidism

The two most common causes of hypothyroidism are iodine deficiency and chronic thyroiditis. Although iodine deficiency is rare in Europe and the United States, it is very common throughout the rest of the world. See Chapter 12 for a more detailed discussion of this problem. As mentioned earlier in this chapter, chronic thyroiditis is an inherited condition that is diagnosed by checking the levels of thyroid autoantibodies in the blood.

In addition to these two causes of hypothyroidism, many other reasons for people becoming hypothyroid exist. The causes detailed in the following sections are normally ruled out before your doctor starts treating your condition with thyroid hormone replacement.

Removal of the thyroid

If your thyroid is removed because of cancer or an infection, or in the course of treatment for hyperthyroidism (see Chapter 6), you usually become hypothyroid. Only if some tissue is left behind does the thyroid possibly continue to function, although it's unlikely to produce enough thyroid hormones to meet your needs.

Absence of brain hormones

Anything that destroys the *hypothalamus* (the part of the brain that secretes *thyrotrophin-releasing hormone (TRH)*) or the *pituitary gland* at the base of the brain (which secretes thyroid-stimulating hormone (TSH)) produces *central hypothyroidism* – hypothyroidism originating in the control centre of the body, the brain. A trauma, infection, or infiltration (a replacement of brain tissue with other tissue, which can occur when a patient has cancer) can cause this type of destruction. The same result can occur if the pituitary is exposed to a destructive treatment that prevents the production and release of TSH, such as radiotherapy (radiation treatment) to the area of the pituitary gland.

If hypothyroidism is caused by a problem with the hypothalamus or pituitary, some of the signs and symptoms associated with chronic (autoimmune) thyroiditis are not found. In particular, hoarseness and a thickened tongue occur in autoimmune hypothyroidism but not in hypothyroidism associated with a lack of brain hormones. In addition, the thyroid is not usually enlarged in this instance, because TSH is not stimulating it (because the brain isn't making TSH). Also, the person's hair and skin are not coarse in this situation (but they are if the patient has autoimmune hypothyroidism).

Symptoms that result from a lack of other pituitary hormones also help to differentiate central hypothyroidism from failure of the thyroid gland. These include fine wrinkling of the skin of the face and a more pronounced loss of underarm, pubic, and facial hair.

Foods that cause hypothyroidism

Interestingly, many common foods can cause hypothyroidism if you eat them in sufficient quantities, especially if you have an iodine deficiency. These foods are called *goitrogens* because they can trigger enlargement of the thyroid (a goitre) as well as hypothyroidism. They block the conversion of T4 hormone to T3, the active form of thyroid hormone (refer to Chapter 3). Among the more common foods that cause this condition are:

- Almonds
- Brussel sprouts
- Cabbage
- Cauliflower
- Corn
- Kale
- Turnips

If your condition is due to consuming these foods, simply removing them from your diet cures your hypothyroidism. Your thyroid takes three to six weeks to return to normal after you stop eating these foods.

Drugs that cause hypothyroidism

Many different medications cause hypothyroidism in the same way as the goitrogens listed in the previous section; they block the conversion of T4 to T3. The drugs most likely to trigger this condition include:

- Adrenal steroids like prednisone and hydrocortisone, which treat inflammation

> ✔ Amiodarone, a heart drug
>
> ✔ Antithyroid drugs like propylthiouricil and carbimazole (see Chapter 6)
>
> ✔ Lithium, for psychiatric treatment
>
> ✔ Propranolol, a beta-blocker (see Chapter 6)

Coexisting autoimmune diseases

Occasionally, someone with an autoimmune thyroid disease has other autoimmune conditions, many of which involve other glands of the body. For example, diabetes mellitus Type 1 sometimes occurs together with an autoimmune thyroid disease. The cause of the diabetes is the autoimmune destruction of the insulin-producing cells of the pancreas. Another example is Addison's disease, in which autoimmune destruction of the adrenal gland takes place. Addison's disease is associated with severe fatigue and low blood pressure and is especially important to identify; giving thyroid hormone without adrenal hormone to such a patient is dangerous as they can collapse due to lack of adrenal hormones.

Autoimmune destruction of the ovaries in women, or the testicles in men, may also occur when someone has autoimmune thyroiditis. The result for women is failure to menstruate, and for men infertility and impotence.

Another gland that is sometimes affected by an autoimmune disease is the *parathyroid* (which actually consists of four parathyroid glands) sitting behind the thyroid in the neck. Loss of parathyroid function results in low blood calcium and the possibility of severe muscle spasms and psychological changes.

Some autoimmune diseases that affect the joints of the body are found together with autoimmune thyroiditis. Rheumatoid arthritis is the most common example, but other diseases such as *Sjögren's syndrome* and *systemic lupus erythematosus* are also diagnosed.

Lastly, the blood disease called pernicious anaemia is an autoimmune disease that accompanies autoimmune thyroiditis on occasion. In this condition, cells of the stomach that produce acid are destroyed by autoimmunity. The patient is unable to absorb vitamin B12 and develops an anaemia (low blood count) along with symptoms in the nervous system.

On occasion, when these diseases occur together, treatment of one of them treats the other at the same time. For example, treating the hypothyroidism with thyroid hormone may greatly improve the diabetes.

Diagnosing Severe Hypothyroidism

Hypothyroidism is rarely seen in its severest form in the United Kingdom – severe hypothyroidism is known as *thyroid storm* – but if the disease is left untreated and total thyroid failure occurs, the patient may die. The clinical picture that develops is one of extreme worsening of the signs and symptoms described earlier in the chapter. The skin becomes extremely dry and coarse, and the person's hair falls out. The person may lose all their eyebrows (and sometimes their eyelashes), and their body temperature may fall to a low level. The person becomes less and less active and may lapse into a coma (called *myxoedema coma*) that can last for many days until they die of heart failure or infection. (The infection or heart disease may precipitate the myxoedema coma in the first place in an elderly person with very low thyroid function.)

Because food is absorbed extremely slowly in severe hypothyroidism, treatment may require injections of thyroid hormones (described in the next section). (See Chapter 6 for more on thyroid storm.)

Treating Hypothyroidism

The treatment of hypothyroidism was once considered very complicated, but is now fairly simple after a diagnosis is made. However, a number of newer thoughts on the subject are worth considering as you and your doctor discuss treatment.

Taking the right hormones

People with hypothyroidism due to chronic thyroiditis, or because of the removal of the thyroid, have to take daily thyroid hormone replacement pills.

The first treatment to replace absent thyroid hormone came from the thyroids of animals and was called *desiccated thyroid*. For many decades, this type of hormone replacement was the only treatment available.

When making T4 hormone in the laboratory became possible, T4 (also called *L-thyroxine*) quickly replaced desiccated thyroid. This change was made for several reasons. First, the amount of hormone in a given animal's thyroid differs from animal to animal, so the dose delivered varies considerably. Second, desiccated thyroid contains both T4 and T3 in amounts that are significantly different from the way it's secreted by the normal thyroid gland (check out Chapter 3).

For many years, doctors suspected that generic forms of thyroid hormone replacement pills (ones without a brand name) did not consistently provide a known level of the hormone, so doctors recommended brand name products so each person received exactly the same name of tablet with each prescription. Recent studies show that generic thyroid hormone has the same potency as brand name thyroid hormone and is, of course, much cheaper.

Because 80 per cent of the T3 thyroid hormone in your body comes from the conversion of T4 into T3 (at sites other than the thyroid), doctors usually give T4 alone and the body normally takes care of producing the T3 it needs. Some recent studies show that when the human thyroid releases thyroid hormone, about 10 per cent is T3 (and the rest is T4). As a result, researchers wonder whether some people with hypothyroidism who take a mixture of T3 and T4 replacement hormone may feel better than those given T4 alone. Several studies involving combination treatment with T4 and T3 have been published in medical journals, including the *Journal of Clinical Endocrinology and Metabolism* (the foremost peer reviewed publication in the field of Endocrinology), as well as the *Journal of the American Medical Association*. According to the British Thyroid Association (see Appendix B), the overall conclusion from these recent studies is that people taking combination therapy do not do any better than those taking T4 alone. In fact, some studies show a detrimental effect on psychological function with combination therapy.

However, doctors are keeping an open mind about combination therapy, and as new evidence becomes available, current opinions may change.

At present, however, almost all people in the world who are currently receiving replacement thyroid hormone to treat hypothyroidism are taking T4 alone. But people have every right to receive a treatment they wish to try, as long as it's legal. So, if you're receiving T4 and still do not feel right, ask your doctor about taking both T3 and T4 together. Your doctor can review the latest evidence and consider whether or not the combination is likely to help you.

If the cause of your hypothyroidism is something other than autoimmune failure of your thyroid, or removal of your thyroid, the underlying cause is also dealt with at the same time as you take thyroid hormone replacement. For example, if you have a pituitary tumour that is responsible for a loss of TSH, the tumour is treated, and any other hormones that are deficient are replaced in addition to thyroid hormones. If your hypothyroidism is caused by a drug or food, removal of that drug or food usually cures the condition. However, sometimes you must continue to take the culprit drug, if no suitable alternative exists. In this case, your doctor prescribes thyroid hormone replacement to alleviate the hypothyroidism for as long as you continue to take the medication.

Getting the right amount

The amount of thyroid hormone that you receive is determined using a TSH test (assuming that central hypothyroidism is not the diagnosis). Depending on the particular laboratory doing the test, the TSH level is usually 0.3–4.5 µU/ml (microunits per millilitre). (Check out Chapter 4 for more on this test.)

Keep in mind that some doctors question whether this measure actually is the normal range for TSH. Ten per cent of the population tests positive for thyroid autoantibodies and probably has autoimmune thyroid disease. Most of these people are not given the diagnosis of hypothyroidism. When a laboratory creates a normal range, it tests several hundred or more people who are considered free of thyroid disease, usually because they have no signs or symptoms. The laboratory measures their TSH and states that 'this is the range for TSH in the normal population.' Are they really measuring a normal population when one of every 10 people tested may have an undiagnosed thyroid disease?

Some patients do not feel normal with a TSH between the normal range, and feel better when given enough thyroid hormone to lower their TSH to below the usual range.

If you are receiving treatment for hypothyroidism and don't feel right on your current dose of replacement thyroid hormone, ask your doctor to check your TSH. Then ask the doctor whether they are willing to prescribe more thyroid hormone to lower your TSH further. Some endocrinologists believe that complete wellbeing is only restored when T4 levels are towards the upper limit of normal, and the TSH level is slightly suppressed below the normal range. This dosage is something you need to discuss with your doctor so you can aim for a result that minimises risks of side effects while at the same time optimising your metabolic rate so problems such as weight gain are less problematic.

Tinkering with thyroxine doses yourself is never a good idea. Excess thyroxine is potentially toxic and can cause rapid pulse, palpitations, heart rhythm abnormalities such as atrial fibrillation and even angina, not to mention diarrhoea, tremor, headache, sweating, muscle weakness, and insomnia.

Another important point is that hypothyroidism is not necessarily permanent. Up to 25 per cent of people with autoimmune hypothyroidism may return to normal thyroid function at a later date. The reason is that production of the autoantibodies that block the action of TSH may decline over time.

If your autoimmune hypothyroidism has gone on for several years, ask your doctor if you can stop the thyroid hormone replacement for four to six weeks to see whether or not your TSH remains low. (Do not stop taking your hormone replacement without your doctor's supervision.)

On the other hand, a thyroid gland that is failing due to autoimmune thyroiditis goes through several levels of failure. At first, you may need little thyroid hormone to replace what you're missing. With time, more of your thyroid tissue may fail or the antibodies that block TSH may increase, and you will need more. Seeing your doctor on a regular basis to check for this increasing (or decreasing) failure of the thyroid is important.

After your thyroid function stabilises, see your doctor every six months or every year to have your TSH level checked and your dosage of thyroid hormone altered if necessary. These checkups are important because you may not feel different in yourself, even if your thyroid function gradually declines.

Testing hormone levels

It takes about four weeks for a change in your dose of replacement thyroid hormone to make a difference in your lab tests. If your dose is changed, you're normally retested regularly to ensure that you're on the correct dose.

Chapter 6

Taming an Overactive Thyroid

*H*yperthyroidism refers to the excessive production of thyroid hormones. The condition leads to many signs and symptoms that suggest your body is, in effect, speeding up.

Hyperthyroidism is fairly common. Each year, about 1 new case is diagnosed per 1,000 people, most of whom are women. That number adds up to more than 60,000 new cases in the United Kingdom every year, because the United Kingdom's population is at least 60 million.

Most people with hyperthyroidism (about 80 per cent) have an autoimmune disorder called Graves' disease, which this chapter discusses in detail. As well as causing signs and symptoms of hyperthyroidism, Graves' disease also affects the eyes and skin. These abnormalities are all bound together by the fact that they result from autoimmunity. (Refer to Chapter 4 for a discussion of 'Thyroid autoantibodies'.) In some circumstances, a person has hyperthyroidism but no eye or skin disease, and blood tests show no evidence of autoimmunity. These people do not have an autoimmune disorder, but their hyperthyroid state produces the same medical picture as if they had Graves' disease.

This chapter shows you how to recognise hyperthyroidism, tells you about the treatment options and the possible complications that may occur as a result of the treatment or the disease itself. Many people believe that if you have hyperthyroidism, you're lucky because the condition makes weight control or weight loss easier. This chapter shows you why that thinking is seriously flawed.

Picturing Hyperthyroidism

Tammy is the mother of Stacy and Karen, who have recently learned that they have autoimmune thyroiditis and hypothyroidism, respectively (refer to Chapter 5). Tammy is a very active person, but lately she has noticed a lot of things wrong with her, and they are getting worse.

Tammy feels warm all the time, and her skin is moist. A few months ago, she lost some weight without trying and was delighted, but the weight loss has continued despite the fact that she has a really strong appetite and is eating more than usual. She often feels her heart racing, which makes her very nervous. She notices that her hands shake when she just sits quietly. She goes to the bathroom more frequently than usual, both to urinate and to open her bowels.

The changes in Tammy are not lost on her husband, Patrick, or her daughters. They notice that she is constantly staring at them, though when they question her, she denies it. Patrick, in the course of giving her a massage to help her relax, notices a bump on the front of her neck that was not there before. Tammy's family insists that she see their family doctor.

The GP asks a number of questions and does a physical examination. He discovers that Tammy's thyroid is enlarged, and he finds a skin abnormality on her lower legs. He tells the family that Tammy almost certainly has hyperthyroidism due to Graves' disease. The final diagnosis requires only some confirmatory blood tests, and the outcome of those tests is so certain that the doctor prescribes Tammy medication to calm her heart rate down, as well as referring her to an endocrinologist at the local hospital for specialist advice.

The tests confirm the diagnosis. Tammy sees the specialist and immediately starts taking an antithyroid pill once a day. By the end of three weeks, she feels better, and after eight weeks, she is her old self. She is a bit disappointed when the pounds start coming back on, but she feels so good that she returns to her health club and sheds several of them in no time. Patrick is, of course, delighted to have his wife back at moderate instead of high speed. Now he wants to visit a London theatre in the West End as he knows she would not sit through a play in her previous condition.

Listing the Signs and Symptoms of Hyperthyroidism

Hyperthyroidism, whether caused by Graves' disease or another condition, produces consistent signs and symptoms that affect every part of your body.

The major abnormalities are described in the following sections, grouped according to the organ system of the body that is affected.

The body generally

Hyperthyroidism can raise your body temperature persistently high. You may lose weight despite an increased appetite. The weight loss is due to the loss of lean body tissue like muscle, not due to a loss of fat. In rare cases, however, you may gain weight because you're eating so many calories. Hyperthyroidism can cause you to feel weak. You may feel enlarged lymph glands all over your body (for example in your neck, armpits, and groin), because Graves' disease is an autoimmune disease and the lymph system is a key player in autoimmunity. Your tonsils, which are part of the lymph system, are also enlarged.

Other possible reasons for enlargement of the lymph glands can be more serious than Graves' disease, so if you experience this symptom, see your doctor.

The thyroid

When Graves' disease is the cause of hyperthyroidism, your thyroid is enlarged in a symmetrical way and the entire gland is firm. When a single overactive nodule (a lump on your thyroid) is to blame for hyperthyroidism, that nodule is large, but it often causes the rest of the gland to shrink. (Head to Chapter 7 for a discussion on nodules.) When a multinodular goitre is responsible (see Chapter 9), you can feel many lumps and bumps on your thyroid.

If you put your hand over an enlarged thyroid, you can often feel a buzzing sensation, called a thrill, which results from the great increase in blood flow through the overactive gland. You can also hear the thrill with a stethoscope; the sound is called a bruit (pronounced _brooeee_).

The skin and hair

Hyperthyroidism can make your hands feel warm and moist, and they may appear red. You may experience a loss of skin pigmentation (a condition called vitiligo) in places, which is another sign of autoimmunity. Other areas of your skin may appear darker. Sometimes hair changes, too, becoming fine, straight, and unable to hold a curl.

The heart

Hyperthyroidism can cause a rapid pulse, which you feel as heart palpitations. The first sign of Graves' disease is sometimes *atrial fibrillation*, an irregular heart rhythm. If the person is older and already has heart disease, hyperthyroidism can induce heart failure. The condition can also bring on heart pain (angina) or make pre-existing angina worse because your heart is working hard, beating too rapidly. You may also experience shortness of breath.

The nervous system and muscles

If you have hyperthyroidism, your fingers have a fine tremor when you hold your hands out. The loss of muscle tissue leads to weakness. Your reflexes are increased and some people find it impossible to sit still. The mental changes associated with hyperthyroidism are discussed in Chapter 2. Basically, if you're hyperthyroid, most likely you're anxious, nervy, you don't sleep as much as you used to, and you have rapidly changing emotions, from exhilaration to depression.

The reproductive system

Hyperthyroidism can cause a decrease in fertility because it interferes with ovulation in women. Menstrual flow is decreased as well and may even stop temporarily until treatment brings your thyroid function back towards normal.

The stomach and intestines

If you are hyperthyroid, food moves more quickly through your intestines than it used to, and you have more frequent bowel movements or even diarrhoea. You may experience nausea and vomiting.

The urinary system

As blood flows more quickly through your body, more blood passes through your kidneys that are filtering out more urine than normal. As a result, you need to visit the bathroom more frequently. In turn, you feel more thirsty than usual.

The eyes

Any form of hyperthyroidism results in changes to the eyes, most of which are reversible. Your upper eyelids may look pulled up higher so that you can see more of the white above each pupil; this feature makes you appear as if you're staring and pop-eyed. When you are asked to look down, your upper eyelid may not follow your eye, which exposes even more of the white. This disorder is called lid lag.

Graves' disease can also cause more serious eye problems, which are not reversible. These problems are discussed later in this chapter.

Confirming a Diagnosis of Hyperthyroidism

The signs and symptoms described in the previous section usually lead to a conclusive diagnosis of hyperthyroidism, which is confirmed by blood tests. Among the lab findings that can lead to a diagnosis, the following are most important:

- The levels of both free T4 and free T3 (thyroid hormones) in your blood are elevated, and the thyroid-stimulating hormone (TSH) level is suppressed (refer to Chapter 4). The definitive tests for hyperthyroidism are the TSH and the free T4. In 1 per cent of people with hyperthyroidism, a raised level of free T3 can occur, with a normal level of free T4; this condition is called T3 thyrotoxicosis (see the section 'Recognising Other Causes of Hyperthyroidism' later in this chapter).

- If Graves' disease is the cause of hyperthyroidism, the levels of peroxidase autoantibody and antithyroglobulin autoantibody are elevated (check out Chapter 4).

- Your blood glucose (sugar) level is elevated because your body is absorbing food so rapidly.

- You may have insulin resistance, and diabetes may develop or become worse if it's already present. (Diabetes improves after the hyperthyroidism is treated.)

- Blood tests of your liver function (such as the alkaline phosphatase and bilirubin levels in the blood) are sometimes elevated.

- Blood tests for cholesterol and other fats are often lower than normal as you are burning up so much extra energy.

Determining Whether Graves' Disease Is the Culprit

Most cases of hyperthyroidism result from Graves' disease, which is an autoimmune condition. Graves' disease is most common in females and occurs 10 to 20 times more often in women than in men. Symptoms tend to start between the ages of 30 and 60, but they can occur at any age. Graves' disease consists of any one or all of three parts:

- ✔ Hyperthyroidism
- ✔ Eye disease
- ✔ Skin disease

Most of the signs and symptoms of Graves' disease are the result of hyperthyroidism, which in turn results from the excessive production of thyroid hormones. Doctors can distinguish Graves' disease from other forms of hyperthyroidism because blood tests identify autoimmunity. In addition to the symptoms of hyperthyroidism detailed earlier in this chapter, autoimmunity can lead to eye and skin disease.

Causes of Graves' disease

About 10 per cent of the world's population has thyroid autoantibodies (refer to Chapter 5), and these autoantibodies can lead to both hypothyroidism (underactive thyroid function) and hyperthyroidism. These conditions occur because some autoantibodies suppress the thyroid, while others stimulate it. If you have Graves' disease, the stimulating antibodies are in control in your body. Just why this change happens isn't clear, but researchers have a number of theories, including the following:

- ✔ The body makes many cells to prevent foreign tissue from invading and other cells that recognise the body's own tissue. When someone has an autoimmune disorder, their body may have lost the cells meant to prevent other cells from reacting against the body's own tissue.

- ✔ Invading organisms such as viruses may share characteristics of normal body tissue. When the body creates antibodies to fight the invaders, those antibodies may react against normal tissue as well.

- ✔ Certain drugs can change the immunity of the body so it reacts against itself. These drugs are used in the treatment of hepatitis and leukaemia, for example, and their effect is to activate or increase immunity. As a side effect, they may activate thyroid-stimulating immunity.

✔ Women, especially, may have genes that promote autoimmunity. The frequent occurrence of Graves' disease in mothers, daughters, and sisters confirms the genetic association (head to Chapter 17).

✔ When the thyroid is injured, for example by a viral illness, it releases chemicals into the blood that are not normally found there. The protective immunity cells may make antibodies against those chemicals, which then react back at the thyroid.

✔ If someone with a large thyroid gland (such as a multinodular goitre; see Chapter 9) that isn't making enough thyroid hormone takes iodine tablets, that person may undergo a sudden production of a lot of thyroid hormone that leads to hyperthyroidism.

✔ Stress can produce a rapid heart rate, sweating, and other signs similar to hyperthyroidism. Its role in the onset of hyperthyroidism is unclear.

Signs and symptoms specific to Graves' disease

The eye and skin problems associated with Graves' disease are sometimes apparent even when a person has no overt symptoms of hyperthyroidism. Sometimes these eye and skin conditions progress even after hyperthyroidism is under control. Severe forms of both these problems are rare, but thyroid eye disease can lead to blindness.

Thyroid eye disease

Thyroid eye disease, called *infiltrative ophthalmopathy* or *exophthalmos*, is present in almost all people with Graves' disease. Minor changes are found in up to 50 per cent of people, increasing to 90 per cent if all are investigated with ultrasound of the eye area. For some reason, smokers are more likely to develop ophthalmopathy than non-smokers. Usually, the condition is mild and does not progress after hyperthyroidism is controlled. Sometimes – in no more than 5 per cent of people with Graves' disease – the condition does progress despite controlling the hyperthyroidism.

Someone with thyroid eye disease presents a clear-cut clinical picture. The eye, with its muscles and coverings, sits in a bony hollow within the skull, called the orbit. When eye disease is present, the skin covering the eye and the muscles within the orbit are swollen and puffy. Since limited room is available within the orbit, the swollen skin and muscles are forced to push forward. Usually both eyes are affected, but the disease can start or progress more rapidly on one side than the other. If your eye is pushed forward far enough, your eyelids cannot close fully. The result is irritation and redness of the eyeball.

The optic nerve that carries the visual signal to your brain is stretched and sometimes damaged by thyroid eye disease, as is the back of the eye, the retina, where your eye focuses what it sees. Swelling can also compromise the blood supply to these tissues.

Additionally, the eye muscles do not function properly, so that your eyes do not move together; you may experience double vision as a result. Someone with Graves' ophthalmopathy may first notice mild symptoms such as excess tears, intolerance of light and grittiness, or more severe symptoms such as eye pain, double vision, and reduced vision. Occasionally, the end result of this damage is blindness but this state is rare.

When the eye muscles of a person with thyroid eye disease are examined under a microscope, large numbers of autoimmune cells appear (similar to what is seen in the thyroid itself).

Treatment of thyroid eye disease is usually carried out in steps; severe measures are used only when milder measures fail. First, local measures like eye drops are given to treat the inflammation. If that fails to cure the problem, oral steroids are given to reduce your immunity. Other drugs that suppress immunity are also available.

Severe cases of thyroid eye disease usually respond to irradiation of the muscles in the orbit. If that treatment does not work or the case is severe enough, a surgeon can remove bone from the orbit; thus, decompressing the tissues.

A few simple measures can help improve eye symptoms, such as:

- Avoiding dust
- Wearing sunglasses
- Using artificial teardrops (from chemists or on prescription from your doctor)
- Raising the head of your bed (to reduce swelling when lying flat at night)
- Wearing eye protector pads while you sleep

Thyroid skin disease

Thyroid skin disease – known medically by unpronounceable names such as *pretibial myxoedema* and *thyroid acropachy* – is seen even less often than thyroid eye disease and is very severe in only 1–2 per cent of people with Graves' disease.

Pretibial myxoedema is an abnormal thickening of the skin, usually in the front of the lower leg. Raised patches of skin are pink in appearance. The skin problems may last for several months or longer, then gradually improve. If they become severe, they may respond to steroid creams applied under tight dressings.

With thyroid acropachy, a person's fingers become wider, and they may experience arthritic damage to the joints of the fingers. Fortunately, these lesions usually cause only unsightly fingers and no symptoms. People with these symptoms are not given any particular treatment.

Recognising Other Causes of Hyperthyroidism

Although the vast majority of people with hyperthyroidism have Graves' disease, about 20 per cent do not. The others may have one of several other conditions that lead to the increased production of free T4 and T3 (thyroid hormones). The treatment of these conditions may differ from treatment of Graves' disease, so recognising them is important.

Factitious (false) hyperthyroidism occurs when a person is consuming large amounts of thyroid hormone without a doctor's knowledge. Usually some kind of psychological disturbance or a misguided attempt to lose weight causes this behaviour. The way to distinguish between this cause and other causes of hyperthyroidism is to check the size of the thyroid gland; someone with factitious hyperthyroidism has a small thyroid gland. The gland is suppressed by the large amount of thyroid hormone. If a radioactive iodine uptake is done (refer to Chapter 4), the person's thyroid gland won't absorb a great deal of the iodine.

A large thyroid with many nodules that is exposed to a lot of iodine may trigger hyperthyroidism (see Chapter 9). Sometimes, a single nodule may produce excessive amounts of thyroid hormone and cause the rest of the thyroid to shrink. These conditions are felt by a doctor and confirmed by an ultrasound study or a thyroid scan (refer to Chapter 4).

Occasionally, the thyroid produces large amounts of T3 but normal or even low levels of T4. This condition is called *T3 thyrotoxicosis*. T3 thyrotoxicosis is an autoimmune condition and produces the same signs and symptoms and is treated in exactly the same way as Graves' disease (which is associated with a high free T4 level). This condition is really just Graves' disease with a predominance of T3. Doctors don't yet know why T3 is elevated in these cases rather than T4. If you have the signs and symptoms of hyperthyroidism but your free T4 level is normal or even low, ensure that your doctor measures your T3 level.

A condition called *subacute thyroiditis* (see Chapter 11) may cause the release of a lot of thyroid hormone from the thyroid and briefly cause hyperthyroidism. In the condition, the thyroid is usually tender, and the hyperthyroidism does not last.

A certain (not very common) type of tumour called a *choriocarcinoma*, which arises from the placental tissue between a foetus and its mother, produces a lot of a hormone that stimulates the thyroid. This hormone, human chorionic gonadotrophin, can be measured in the blood.

Finally, *central hyperthyroidism* is also possible, although it occurs much less frequently than Graves' disease. Too much thyrotrophin-releasing hormone from the hypothalamus in the brain, or too much thyroid-stimulating hormone (TSH) from the pituitary gland in the brain (often as a result of a tumour) causes central hyperthyroidism. In this condition, the person's TSH level is high (whereas with Graves' disease this level is low). The person may experience symptoms of increased pressure in the brain, such as headache or loss of part of the visual field.

Your doctor shouldn't have difficulty differentiating Graves' disease from any of the conditions discussed in this section, especially if the doctor looks for signs that your eyes and skin are changing, and requests tests that check for thyroid autoantibodies.

Choosing the Best Treatment for Graves' Disease

The treatment of Graves' disease has evolved over the years as doctors and researchers have come to understand it better and additional tools have become available. As soon as doctors understood that the thyroid was responsible for the excessive production of thyroid hormones, the obvious response was to cut out the offending tissue. This produced an era of great thyroid surgeons, along with a lot of unexpected problems that are described in the next section. Around 1950, the administration of radioactive iodine (RAI) started to replace surgery and, although it cures many people, the treatment brings its own difficulties. Finally, antithyroid drugs became available.

Each form of treatment has its pros and cons. Interestingly, doctors in Europe generally prefer treating with antithyroid pills, while doctors in the United States are more likely to choose radioactive iodine. The following sections explain the advantages and disadvantages of each form of treatment. As a rule, however, research shows that each form of treatment, whether antithyroid drugs, radioactive iodine, or surgery, is associated with similar improvements in quality of life and similar degrees of patient satisfaction, so the choice often comes down to the doctor or patient's preference. The effectiveness of any treatment is initially monitored by measuring levels of free thyroxine (T4) as low levels of thyroid-stimulating hormone (TSH) often persist for many months despite the proper treatment.

Thyroid surgery

Thyroid surgery involves the removal of all or part of the thyroid gland. Surgery quickly reduces the symptoms of hyperthyroidism as it removes the source of those symptoms – the thyroid that was producing too much hormone.

With the availability of non-surgical treatments, surgery is rarely done today for hyperthyroidism. Some situations leave surgery as the only choice, such as the following:

✔ The patient refuses to take radioactive iodine and develops an allergy or a bad reaction to antithyroid pills (or simply fails to take them).

✔ The thyroid gland is extremely large, which means that radioactive iodine or antithyroid pills are less effective.

✔ The diagnosis of hyperthyroidism is made during pregnancy and is not properly controlled with antithyroid drugs, causing problems for the mother or the foetus. (Surgery is okay if done between the third and sixth month of pregnancy.)

✔ The thyroid has nodules that suggest a possible cancer.

One reason why surgery is not often used to treat thyroid conditions these days is that surgery carries certain risks:

✔ Any operation requiring anaesthesia involves risk.

✔ Surgery is not safe for someone with severe heart or lung disease.

✔ Surgery is not advisable during the last three months of pregnancy, because it could induce early labour.

✔ Surgery can damage one or both nerves supplying the voice box (*recurrent laryngeal nerves*), which can lead to hoarseness or permanent damage to the voice.

✔ Surgery can damage the *parathyroid glands* that lie behind the thyroid, leading to a severe drop in blood calcium.

✔ Although a surgeon's goal is sometimes to leave enough thyroid tissue to keep the patient's thyroid function normal, low thyroid function may begin immediately after surgery or develop during the next few years. These days, most surgery is designed to remove the whole thyroid gland (total thyroidectomy).

   ✔ If someone has had previous neck surgery, attempting another operation is risky as important nerves and arteries may be tangled up in scar tissue.

   ✔ In people with hyperthyroidism who have only part of their thyroid gland removed during surgery, 10 per cent have a relapse and develop hyperthyroidism again over a period of ten years.

Some specialists believe that surgery releases thyroid antigens (tissue or chemicals to which the body is not normally exposed) into the blood stream and, where a lot of thyroid tissue is left intact, this can worsen the autoimmune condition, possibly resulting in worse eye disease. Whether or not this belief is true is unclear.

For more information about thyroid surgery, see Chapter 13.

Radioactive iodine treatment

In this treatment, a person swallows a capsule containing radioactive iodine (RAI). Because the thyroid uses more iodine than any other organ or gland in the body, the RAI quickly concentrates in the thyroid and releases enough radiation to slowly destroy the overactive thyroid cells.

Radioactive iodine is an ideal solution to the problem of hyperthyroidism. Decades of experience with radioactive iodine have lain to rest a number of the fears surrounding this treatment:

   ✔ Studies report no increase in thyroid cancer in adults who receive RAI, or of cancer elsewhere in the body.

   ✔ Studies report no increase in cases of leukaemia after RAI.

   ✔ RAI does not affect fertility.

   ✔ Children of mothers who previously received RAI have normal thyroid function and no congenital defects at birth (though RAI is never given during a pregnancy). These children can, however, still develop Graves' disease later in life because it is hereditary.

In addition, RAI is inexpensive and avoids the risks of surgery. But RAI does have its share of drawbacks:

   ✔ RAI is not suitable for a pregnant woman because the drug crosses the placenta and enters the baby's thyroid, possibly destroying it.

   ✔ RAI is not suitable for use in small children (younger than teenagers) because of the incidence of thyroid cancer when small children (whose thyroid gland is still developing) are exposed to it. (For example, thyroid cancer was rampant among children exposed to RAI outside the Russian nuclear plant at Chernobyl.)

✔ Finding the exact dose to cure the hyperthyroidism but leave the patient with normal thyroid function is impossible. If too little RAI is used, another treatment is needed. Most patients given enough RAI to cure their hyperthyroidism do eventually become hypothyroid (usually within three to six months) and need to take thyroid hormone replacement for life. The likelihood of developing hypothyroidism RAI is low if the hyperthyroidism is due to toxic multinodular goitre, or to a toxic nodule, however.

✔ If RAI causes hypothyroidism, patients may experience three unusual symptoms: joint aches, stiffness, and headaches. The headaches are possibly due to swelling of the pituitary gland.

✔ By slowly destroying the thyroid, RAI releases a large amount of thyroid antigens into the patient's circulation (similar to the situation with surgery), which may greatly increase autoimmunity and make eye disease worse.

✔ People receiving RAI need follow-up blood tests for years to monitor for the development of hypothyroidism.

After RAI is given, it takes about three weeks to start having an effect, and the maximal effect occurs about two months after treatment. These timeframes can vary depending on how large the gland is when the treatment occurs, however.

Antithyroid pills

In the United Kingdom, there are two antithyroid pills used to control hyperthyroidism, propylthiouracil (PTU) and carbimazole. Both pills block the production of thyroid hormones, but propylthiouracil also blocks the conversion of T4 to T3, giving it a theoretical advantage over carbimazole. This advantage doesn't seem to matter much in practise unless you are trying to control the hyperthyroidism very rapidly and, overall, carbimazole is more widely used in the United Kingdom.

A major advantage of these pills is that, unlike surgery or radioactive iodine, they help to treat all complications of Graves' disease, including eye disease, as they reduce autoimmunity. Also, given in correct dosages, they do not lead to hypothyroidism.

When either drug is given, the patient usually starts to feel better after three weeks, and the hyperthyroidism is controlled within six weeks. Then, it is important to monitor the patient's free T4 level at least every six to eight weeks, because treatment can lower T4 into the hypothyroid range.

Two different treatment regimens are used:

- ✔ A titration regime that adjusts doses up and down to try to achieve a normal (euthyroid) state.

- ✔ A block-replace regime in which the antithyroid drug is designed to totally block thyroid, with T4 replaced as a tablet. This regime has the advantage of avoiding hypothyroidism and the need for frequent blood tests to check for hypothyroidism. This method is not suitable during pregnancy.

Neither regime has a clear advantage over the other in terms of outcome. Research suggests that the best length of time for someone to receive the titration regime is 12–18 months, and for the block-replace regime, 6–12 months. People often relapse when treatment is stopped, however. On average, around one-third of people taking antithyroid pills remain under control after they stop taking the propylthiouracil or carbimazole. The people most likely to achieve remission with one of these regimes are those with mild disease and small goitres. For the other two-thirds, the symptoms of hyperthyroidism recur after the pills are stopped. These people can choose to continue on antithyroid drugs or to receive another treatment – either surgery or RAI.

Most people taking an antithyroid drug start on 15–40 mg (milligrams) of carbimazole once a day, while initial doses of propylthiouracil range from 200–400 mg per day divided into three daily doses. As thyroid function returns to normal, after 4–8 weeks, the doctor decides which of the two regimes to use. In the titration regime, the daily dose of drug is gradually reduced to a maintenance dose of 5–15 mg per day for carbimazole, or 50–150 mg per day for propylthiouracil. Regular blood tests help to decide what the best maintenance dose is for an individual person. If the block-replace regime is used, then thyroid hormone replacement is simply added in and the antithyroid drug is kept at its previous higher level.

Like surgery and RAI, antithyroid drugs carry some risks. The major risk is that they can cause a reduction in white blood cells and even, very rarely, a complete lack of white blood cell production (a condition called *agranulocytosis*). If 10,000 people take an antithyroid drug for one year, then just three develop this problem. Although this condition usually occurs within the first three months of treatment, in people taking especially large doses of medication, the condition is occasionally seen later on and at low doses. This problem goes away when the person stops taking the drug.

One way to avoid severe loss of white blood cell production is to have a white cell count done each time you visit your doctor while you are on these pills.

If you are on carbimazole or propylthiouracil and develop a fever, sore throat, mouth ulcers, or other symptoms of infection stop taking the antithyroid drug and see your doctor for an urgent blood test to see whether you just have a cold or whether you've developed a low white blood cell count.

Some people taking antithyroid drugs develop skin rashes and itching. If relatively mild, these symptoms are treated with an antihistamine without having to stop treatment. Alternatively, if you are taking carbimazole your doctor may switch you to propylthiouracil or the other way round.

Another rare side effect of these drugs is the occurrence of liver function abnormalities and even liver damage. If you take one of these drugs, ask your doctor to check your liver function every few surgery visits.

Other helpful medications

A class of pills called beta-blockers can reduce the symptoms of hyperthyroidism without actually treating the condition. Beta-blockers are valuable for controlling the disease while antithyroid pills or radioactive iodine have a chance to work. They are also prescribed by family doctors to reduce symptoms in people with hyperthyroidism who are waiting to see a hospital specialist for the first time. The most commonly used beta-blocker drugs are propranolol and metoprolol, which help to slow the heart, decrease anxiety, and reduce tremor. Because the liver works more quickly to break down these drugs in people with an overactive thyroid, beta-blockers are taken more often than normal – three to four times a day. They are usually continued for a few weeks until the other medications take effect, or are used as preparation for surgery. In fact, beta-blockers are often the only treatment needed for someone with hyperthyroidism due to thyroiditis.

 People with heart failure as a result of severe hyperthyroidism are given different beta-blockers (bisoprolol and carvedilol) as these drugs are licensed for use in heart failure and do not make the condition worse.

Preparations of iodine are also available for use to temporarily block thyroid hormone production and reduce the blood flowing to the thyroid in preparation for surgery.

Treating Other Causes of Hyperthyroidism

People who have hyperthyroidism that isn't caused by Graves' disease may need other treatment options:

- ✔ People with factitious hyperthyroidism are advised to stop taking their thyroid pills and start some form of psychotherapy.

- ✔ A thyroid with one or more nodules that produce too much thyroid hormone responds best to radioactive iodine (RAI); because the nodules are not caused by an autoimmune condition; thus, eliminating the concern about thyroid eye disease lingering after the treatment. In the case of a single nodule causing the hyperthyroidism, the nodule is eliminated with RAI, and the rest of the thyroid often returns to normal function. When single or multiple overactive nodules are present, antithyroid drugs almost never cause a permanent remission.

- ✔ T3 thyrotoxicosis responds to antithyroid medication just like Graves' disease due to excess T4.

- ✔ The hyperthyroid phase of subacute thyroiditis does not last very long. If necessary, the beta-blocker propranolol can control symptoms until the hyperthyroidism subsides.

- ✔ When symptoms are due to a choriocarcinoma making hormones that stimulate the thyroid, the tumour is always removed.

- ✔ A tumour in the brain causing excessive production of thyroid-stimulating hormone must be treated by surgery or radiation therapy.

Surviving Thyroid Storm

Severe hyperthyroidism, known as *thyroid storm*, is a rare condition that is sometimes fatal. The clinical picture is one of extreme signs and symptoms of hyperthyroidism. The person affected has a high fever and a very rapid heartbeat. The person may vomit, have diarrhoea, and often be dehydrated. They may develop heart failure and have a heart rhythm that is difficult to control. The person can lapse into delirium or even a coma.

Fortunately, thyroid storm is rarely seen because hyperthyroidism is almost always diagnosed at a much earlier stage. The condition is sometimes seen when partially controlled hyperthyroidism is complicated with an added infection. When this state does occur, rapid treatment is essential.

This condition is a true medical emergency and admission to intensive care is vital, as the person needs careful management from a physician who is very aware of the treatment of severe hyperthyroidism.

The doctor usually starts a number of treatments all at once. The patient is given fluids, one of the antithyroid drugs (such as propylthiouracil), potassium iodide, steroids, and a beta-blocker like propranolol. This combination of medication can lower the level of T3 hormone to normal in a day, although the patient takes many more days to fully recover.

Chapter 7

Getting the Low-Down on Thyroid Nodules

*I*n some ways, the thyroid is a bit of an annoying gland as it has a tendency to keep forming bumps and growths that are of little or no significance. Even so, these thyroid lumps are always fully evaluated by your specialist just in case they prove cancerous – although thyroid cancer is rarely fatal (see Chapter 8). As this gland causes so much trouble, surgeons often feel that they'd love to simply get rid of the thyroid, similar to the way in which they used to fling out misbehaving tonsils and adenoids. However, the thyroid is so important to our health that they usually do their best to give this bit of 'pain in the neck' tissue a reprieve.

The reason that so much attention is paid to the lumps on your thyroid is the same reason why a piece of property is valuable: location, location, location. If the thyroid gland grew inside your chest or abdomen, all these little growths would never get noticed and would cause few problems. Instead, your thyroid is positioned right up front, where everyone can see and feel it, and provides a lifetime source of work for thyroid specialists – some of whom like to call themselves *thyroidologists*. Most specialists call themselves *endocrinologists*, however, as they also have their work cut out dealing with other misfiring endocrine glands. (An endocrine gland is one that secretes hormones directly into the blood stream rather than into a duct.)

This chapter tells you all you need to know about thyroid lumps and bumps by explaining which types of nodules cause concern and which to safely ignore, as well as what happens if you need to have your lump removed. Most thyroid nodules are minor inconveniences and knowing what to do about them tends to keep them that way.

Discovering a Thyroid Nodule

Kenneth is a 35-year-old man in excellent health. While shaving one day, he notices a bump on the front of his neck that he has not seen before. He ignores it for several months but finally decides that he ought to ask someone to check it out. He goes to his doctor, who does thyroid function tests. His free T4 and thyroid-stimulating hormone (TSH) levels are normal (refer to Chapter 4). His doctor then sends him to a thyroidologist for evaluation.

The thyroidologist asks Kenneth if the lump has grown noticeably and if it causes any trouble when swallowing or breathing. Kenneth answers 'no' to these questions. The specialist then proposes that Kenneth has a *fine needle aspiration biopsy (FNAB)* (check out Chapter 4). When this test is done, the hospital report identifies the lump as a *benign thyroid adenoma*, which means it's not cancerous. Kenneth is told to come back in a year for a re-examination.

A year later, the test shows no change, and the specialist asks him to return a year after that. Kenneth forgets about coming back for re-testing and the consultant's secretary fails to remind him – even so, Kenneth lives happily ever after.

Kenneth's a very good example of the typical case history of a person with a thyroid nodule. He illustrates the unexpected finding of a lump, the tendency to ignore it, and the fact that it generally isn't a problem in the long run.

This case is not meant to detract from the fact that some nodules are diagnosed as cancer and are dealt with promptly. This example simply illustrates the most common course of events.

The thyroid is ordinarily a smooth butterfly-shaped gland (refer to Chapter 3). Whenever something grows that alters that smoothness, the growth is called a *nodule*

A person may have one or several growths on their thyroid, and multiple explanations for why they appear. Physicians identify the various possibilities according to the appearance of the nodule tissue under a microscope. This process is known as the pathological appearance of the tissue. For most purposes, doctors and patients alike just want to know whether the nodule is benign (not cancerous) or malignant (cancerous).

The good news is that most thyroid nodules – 90 per cent or more – are benign.

Evaluating Cancer Risks

A number of facts about a person's thyroid history, signs, and symptoms can help to sway the balance towards or away from a diagnosis of cancer:

- ✔ If a person has many nodules, this suggests that a cancer is not present. Most multinodular thyroids are benign.

- ✔ A most important point in a person's history is previous exposure to radiation. (This exposure doesn't include the use of radioactive iodine in the treatment of hyperthyroidism – go to Chapter 6.) For example, children exposed to radiation from the Chernobyl Nuclear Plant in Russia show a significant increase in thyroid cancer. In this case, multiple nodules do not rule out cancer as almost half the nodules in an irradiated gland are cancerous.

- ✔ A nodule that grows rapidly is probably a cancer, but if it pops up suddenly and is tender, this suggests a haemorrhage. A haemorrhage of this form is not usually a serious problem, but it does cause discomfort.

- ✔ Nodules are found less often in men than women, but are cancerous more often in men, when they are found.

- ✔ Nodules found in children are cancerous more frequently than they are in adults. However, a nodule in a child is still benign more often than it is malignant.

- ✔ Virtually no family or hereditary connection is associated with nodules, either benign or cancerous. The exception is a condition called *multiple endocrine neoplasia* where many members of a family have nodules on several different glands, such as the thyroid, the pancreas, the parathyroids, and the adrenal glands.

- ✔ Symptoms of hoarseness and trouble with swallowing suggest cancer.

- ✔ Finding growths in the neck away from the thyroid suggests cancer that has spread, and those growths are also evaluated by a biopsy.

- ✔ If the thyroid doesn't move freely, it's a sign of fixation that suggests cancer.

Securing a Diagnosis

When a GP sees someone with a thyroid lump, the practitioner asks about associated symptoms, such as difficulty breathing or hoarseness, and examines the neck to check for enlarged lymph nodes. If any of these signs or symptoms are present, the doctor then picks up the phone and arranges immediate referral to a thyroid specialist clinic. Although most people would like 'immediate' to mean the same day, in clinical practice it is usually acceptable for immediate to mean within two weeks. If no other symptoms or signs are present, the doctor takes blood to check the thyroid function and autoantibody status. If this test is normal then the person is also referred as soon as possible to a thyroid specialist clinic so that a nodule that is cancerous is rapidly differentiated from one that is benign. If the thyroid function tests are abnormal, then the person is routinely referred to an endocrinologist. Thyroid function tests that suggest hyperthyroidism (refer to Chapter 6) or hypothyroidism (Chapter 5 covers this condition) usually mean that a thyroid nodule is benign. However, two different conditions can exist within the thyroid at the same time. Therefore, doctors examine a coexisting nodule occasionally to ensure that it's not growing.

Once you reach the thyroid specialist clinic, the team arrange tests to correctly diagnose the nature of the nodule.

The fine needle aspiration cytology

This test is the gold standard for diagnosing a single thyroid nodule. Usually, specialists skip the other tests and go right to this simple, painless, and very specific procedure. A tiny needle is stuck into the nodule, sometimes under the guidance of ultrasound, and cells are removed using suction. A cell pathologist with a special interest in thyroid disease then examines the cells under a microscope (hence the word *cytology*, which means study of cells) to find out whether they are cancerous or benign. When sucking out the cells and any fluid, the doctor notes whether or not the nodule resolves – that is, disappears. If the nodule is a fluid-filled cyst that doesn't fully disappear after aspiration, the remaining lump is aspirated again, and the specimens examined separately. Doctors believe that this test gives the correct diagnosis 94 per cent of the time, with false positive or false negative results occurring in only 6 per cent of cases. To ensure accuracy, a cytology specimen from a non-cystic nodule is only accepted as adequate if it contains six or more groups of at least 10 thyroid follicular cells. If the sample is rejected as not adequate, the fine needle aspiration is repeated to obtain more cells. In this situation, ultrasound guidance allows more accurate targeting of the nodule, which is often quite small. Where results suggest the nodule is from a nodular goitre or due to thyroiditis, a further fine needle aspiration cytology is carried out after three to six months to exclude cancer.

The thyroid ultrasound scan

A *thyroid ultrasound scan* (check out Chapter 4) gives a picture of the entire thyroid and demonstrates if more than one nodule is present. More helpful than that, an ultrasound can distinguish between a solid mass and a cyst. A cyst is a nodule that is filled with fluid or contains some solid tissue. A cyst filled with fluid is usually a benign growth. A cyst that contains some solid tissue is sometimes a cancer. The scan can detect cystic nodules as small as 2mm wide and solid lumps that are only 3mm wide.

A *radioactive iodine uptake and thyroid scan* (refer to Chapter 4) is often not necessary when diagnosing a thyroid nodule. Sometimes, the test is useful to distinguish a nodule that takes up radioactive iodine from one that does not. A nodule can actively concentrate iodine even though the thyroid function tests are normal. A 'warm' nodule takes up radioactive iodine like the rest of the gland. If the nodule concentrates most of the iodine (while the rest of the gland is less active) and the thyroid function tests are elevated, it's a 'hot' nodule. Cancerous nodules are usually 'cold', meaning they do not concentrate the radioactivity. However, most cold nodules are not cancerous.

Figure 7-1 shows the typical appearance of a cold nodule and a hot nodule.

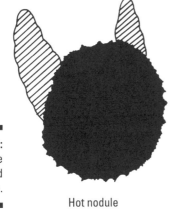 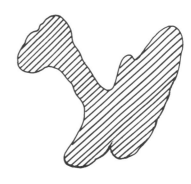

Figure 7-1:
A hot nodule and a cold nodule.

Hot nodule

Cold nodule

In addition, the thyroid scan sometimes shows multiple nodules when only one was seen or felt. Multiple nodules argue against a cancer.

Treating Cancerous Nodules

Every so often, one of these anonymous nodules is diagnosed as a cancer (see Chapter 8), and treatment is necessary. (Sometimes, the tests available to a doctor do not provide a definitive diagnosis, in which case the best step is to treat the nodule as if it is cancerous, just in case.)

The treatment of choice for a cancerous thyroid nodule is surgery. Even benign nodules are sometimes removed surgically if they are unsightly or cause compression or trouble with swallowing.

When surgery is necessary, there are two key requirements:

- ✔ A competent surgeon with plenty of experience in thyroid surgery is vital as potential complications can arise when operating in this part of the neck (see Chapter 13). A general surgeon who carries out only occasional thyroid cases does not usually undertake thyroid surgery for possible cancer, as the cancer is sometimes extensive. Furthermore, the procedure needs to be done successfully the first time around, as a second surgery is much more difficult and complicated due to the formation of scar tissue. For this reason, doctors refer suspected thyroid cancers to a specialist surgeon or endocrinologist who is a member of the local Regional Thyroid Cancer Multidisciplinary Team.

- ✔ An experienced pathologist is also vital to diagnose the type of tissue that the surgeon removes, as surgery proceeds. The pathologist's opinion determines whether the surgeon just removes the lump, or carries out a complete removal of the thyroid (called a *total thyroidectomy*) and removal of lymph nodes in the neck to see if the cancer has spread. This extensive operation is only carried out if the pathologist can give the surgeon a precise diagnosis. Ideally, the final diagnosis of the tissue, made after surgery is complete, doesn't contradict the diagnosis made during the operation.

Dealing with Nodules That Are Non-Cancerous

Hot nodules and benign cysts may require some treatment, but not necessarily surgery. Dealing with the thyroid non-surgically is always preferable because of the potential for surgical complications . Every person has the right to discuss their treatment with their doctor and to request removal of the nodule if they prefer, however. For those who wish to avoid surgery, other treatment choices are available for nodules that are not cancerous.

Hot nodules

A hot nodule produces hyperthyroidism so it needs treatment. One choice is to give the person radioactive iodine (RAI), as is done for Graves' disease (refer to Chapter 6). However, up to 40 per cent of people treated with RAI develop hypothyroidism (underactive thyroid) later in life. Those who do not develop hypothyroidism usually return to normal thyroid function.

A newer treatment that eliminates the hot nodule while not destroying the rest of the thyroid gland is the injection of ethanol (alcohol) into the nodule. This procedure is done several times over several days. Complications include pain in the thyroid area and fever. This treatment is likely to become more and more common as doctors gain experience with it.

Benign cysts

A nodule that is filled with fluid shrinks when a needle is inserted and the fluid is removed. Unfortunately, the cyst often fills right up again. Repeated removal of the fluid sometimes cures the problem. An alternative approach is to inject ethanol into a cyst, the same procedure as injecting into a solid nodule. You can also choose to keep the cyst and leave it alone if you are willing to live with it.

Warm or cold nodules

Nodules that do not produce excessive thyroid hormone and are not cancer are sometimes treated with thyroid hormone in an attempt to shrink the nodule. Little evidence exists to show that this treatment works, however. And, as giving too much thyroid hormone can cause bone loss or an abnormal heartbeat, many endocrinologists no longer recommend thyroid suppression.

Warm and cold nodules are examined every six months or every year. Should the nodule grow, a fine needle biopsy is done again. If the second diagnostic needle aspiration definitely rules out cancer, the nodule is left alone.

Ignoring Small Nodules

Every so often, a test such as an ultrasound of the neck reveals one or more very small nodules on the thyroid. Even the best specialists probably cannot feel a nodule that is less than one centimetre in size. The ultrasound may detect a nodule that is as small as 2–3mm across. One of these tiny, tiny nodules found by accident is referred to as an *incidentaloma* (a thyroid specialist's agonising attempt at humour).

Most consultants monitor these nodules at regular intervals and try to leave them well alone as long as they are not growing in size.

Chapter 8

Coping with Thyroid Cancer

· ·

In This Chapter

▶ Understanding how thyroid cancer starts

▶ Recognising the types of thyroid cancer

▶ Knowing and treating the stages of cancer

▶ Ensuring proper long-term follow-up

· ·

*C*ancer is a word that evokes a number of images, none of which are particularly positive. Although uncommon, people do die of thyroid cancer so this chapter explains what thyroid cancer is, how it grows, how it's treated, and how to follow up after treatment if you or a loved one has thyroid cancer.

The facts and figures in this chapter help put thyroid cancer into perspective. Researchers estimate that as much as 6 per cent of the world's population has cancer of the thyroid gland. Based on this percentage, about 3,600,000 people in the United Kingdom may have evidence of thyroid cancer. Yet in the United Kingdom, out of every one million women, 23 are diagnosed as having thyroid cancer each year, compared with nine new cases for every one million males. In England and Wales, this figure adds up to approximately 900 new cases recognised each year, with 250 recorded deaths. This evidence suggests that the vast majority of people with thyroid cancer live and die without ever knowing that it existed. The cancer is only detected when the thyroid is carefully examined under a microscope which typically occurs after someone notices symptoms, such as a lump.

Thyroid cancer does not appear anywhere near the top of the list of causes of death in the United Kingdom, as it represents only around 1 per cent of all cancers. This figure suggests that compared to most other cancers thyroid cancer is one of the least dangerous. In fact, the long-term outcome is very favourable after treatment, with the 10 year survival rate approaching 90 per cent. No-one wants to have cancer. However, if you had to have cancer, this cancer could seem like one of the better ones to choose. However, between 5–20 per cent of people with thyroid cancer develop recurrences, and up to 15 per cent develop secondaries – where the cancer spreads to other parts of the body. Therefore, this cancer needs to be taken very seriously.

The relatively benign course of most thyroid cancers (see the section 'Identifying the Types of Thyroid Cancer' later in this chapter for the different types of thyroid cancer) makes it difficult to say which treatment is best. Perhaps certain treatments are very effective, or perhaps any number of treatments work just as well because the disease itself is so mild. For this reason, opinions on how to treat thyroid cancer differ among thyroid specialists. Treatment is now more straightforward than it used to be, thanks to the recent development of national, evidence-based guidelines for the management of thyroid cancer in adults. These guidelines are recommendations from the British Thyroid Association and the Royal College of Physicians of London, and are designed to help thyroid specialists select the best treatment for each individual patient. These guidelines are available for download from: www.british-thyroid-association.org

Determining What Causes Thyroid Cancer

John is 40 years old and has noticed a lump in the front of his neck on the left side. His family has no history of thyroid cancer. The lump is painless and moves when he swallows. He doesn't know how long he's had it. John goes to see his doctor, who requests thyroid function tests and finds that the TSH and free T4 are normal. He refers John urgently to the thyroid specialist clinic where a thyroid scan shows that the area of the nodule on John's thyroid does not take up any radioactivity – it's a *cold* nodule. John's endocrinologist then performs a fine needle aspiration biopsy (refer to Chapter 4). The pathologist examines cells from John's thyroid gland under a microscope and diagnoses a papillary cancer, which is the most common type of thyroid cancer.

The thyroid surgeon recommends removing the whole thyroid gland (total thyroidectomy) while carefully retaining the tissue around the parathyroid glands and the recurrent laryngeal nerves that pass along the thyroid. The surgery goes well and no other suspicious nodes or nodules are found during the procedure.

John has no other treatment initially. After three weeks, he has a TSH test. The result is very high indicating that very little thyroid tissue remains in his body (so the pituitary gland produces lots of TSH in a fruitless attempt to increase production of thyroxine hormone). He has another scan that shows no uptake of radioactive iodine except for in a small area of the thyroid tissue that was left intact by the surgeon. John is given a large dose of radioactive iodine to eliminate that small bit of tissue. A follow-up scan shows that all the thyroid tissue is gone. John is placed on thyroid hormone replacement and continues to visit the clinic on a regular basis. John will probably live a normal life span with no further trouble associated with the thyroid cancer other than the periodic visits for follow-up.

John's story is similar to that of most people who develop thyroid cancer, with the cancer first showing itself as a thyroid nodule (check out Chapter 7). Keep in mind that the vast majority of thyroid nodules are not cancerous, however.

Our understanding of why cancer occurs is getting clearer and clearer. We know that certain genes (part of our hereditary make-up) called *oncogenes* cause a cell to grow and divide without controls. Oncogenes exist in all of our cells. Just exactly what switches on certain oncogenes so they are active is not clear, but possibilities include a mistake in cell division (a mutation), some chemical or radiation in the environment, or the effects of a virus.

Human chromosome (our DNA) also contains other genes called *tumour suppressor genes*. Studies suggest that some people lack these tumour suppressor genes and are therefore more likely to develop cancers.

The best-known initiator of thyroid cancer is irradiation (being exposed to radiation), which is the source of many cancers in children living in the area of the Chernobyl nuclear accident in what is now Ukraine. The children drank milk from cows that ate the grass upon which radioactive substances fell – including radioactive iodine, during the reactor core accident. Within just a few years, many of these children had multiple sites of cancer in their thyroid glands. Adults exposed to radioactive iodine also developed thyroid cancer, though not as often as children, as a growing thyroid gland is more sensitive to radioactive damage.

Children who receive neck and face irradiation as an old-fashioned treatment for benign conditions such as acne or enlarged tonsils also develop thyroid cancer. In this case, the cancer occurs as many as 40 years later.

This chapter also discusses cancers of the thyroid that run in families, especially the cancer called *medullary thyroid cancer*.

Identifying the Types of Thyroid Cancer

A pathologist identifies thyroid cancer according to the appearance of the tissue that he or she examines under a microscope. If a nodule is diagnosed as cancer, identifying the particular type of cancer is important, since each one follows a different course. Treatments that work for one type of thyroid cancer may not work at all for a different sort of tumour.

Although you don't need to know how to identify these types of cancer – that's the pathologist's job – a basic understanding of the different types of cancer helps you to know what the future holds if a thyroid cancer is identified. When your doctor tells you the name of that cancer, you have an idea of what to expect.

How a pathologist identifies a cancer

A pathologist looking at thyroid cancer cells under a microscope looks for a number of abnormalities that separate normal tissue from cancerous tissue. He or she has studied thousands of tissue slides and knows the appearance of the tissue when it's found in a person whose clinical course suggests cancer compared with a person who has a benign clinical course. The key things that the pathologist looks for are:

- A malignant appearance to the tissue, which means very large, abnormal looking cells containing abnormal looking parts.

- The presence of even, normal looking tissue in an area where it doesn't belong, which suggests that it has invaded that area – examples are thyroid cells in a lymph gland, in bone, or in the lung.

Cancerous cells that are mature, and closely resemble the type of cell from which it arose, are described as *differentiated*. This is a good sign, as differentiated cancers are normally less aggressive than non-differentiated cancers, which are immature and bear little resemblance to the types of cell from which they arose. Papillary and follicular thyroid cancers are good examples of differentiated cancers.

While the descriptions for each type of thyroid cancer are true for most people with that type of cancer, exceptions do exist. Once in a while, someone with the most aggressive type of thyroid cancer finds that their cancer isn't as aggressive as expected. In the same way, once in a while, a more benign form of thyroid cancer (based on its appearance) takes a more aggressive turn. Medicine is not an exact science.

Papillary thyroid cancer

Papillary thyroid cancer is the most common form of thyroid cancer, accounting for more than 70 per cent of thyroid cancers seen in both adults and children. Fortunately, this form of thyroid cancer also tends to take a benign course, as it is differentiated (meaning it isn't very aggressive). Although the cancer spreads to the local lymph glands in the neck as often as half the time, this spread doesn't seem to make the cancer more aggressive.

The most important characteristics of papillary thyroid cancer are that it

- Rarely spreads away from the neck.
- Is diagnosed most commonly between the ages of 30 and 50.
- Is found in females three times as often as in males.
- Is the thyroid cancer most often associated with radiation exposure.

> ✔ Concentrates radioactive iodine, which is useful if treatment is with radioactive iodine.

> ✔ Is likely to be on a more aggressive course in people over the age of 45, especially if the tumour is larger than 1 centimetre.

> ✔ It's especially mild in younger people, in whom it rarely causes death.

Follicular thyroid cancer

Follicular thyroid cancer makes up another 20 per cent of all thyroid cancers. This cancer is a little more aggressive than papillary cancer, but still usually takes a benign course. It does not tend to spread locally to lymph glands, but goes to bone and the lungs more often than papillary cancer. This cancer's main features are that it

> ✔ Is diagnosed most often between the ages of 40 and 60.

> ✔ Affects females three times as often as males.

> ✔ Concentrates radioactive iodine.

> ✔ Invades blood vessels, accounting for its tendency to go to distant sites.

> ✔ Is usually more aggressive in older people.

Another cancer that follows a course similar to follicular cancer, but has a different appearance under the microscope, is called a *Hurthle cell tumour*. It does not tend to concentrate radioactive iodine, so this is not a useful form of treatment.

Medullary thyroid cancer

Medullary thyroid cancer makes up only about 5–10 per cent of all cancers of the thyroid gland.

This cancer does not arise in the cells that produce thyroid hormones; rather, it arises in another type of cell found in the thyroid, called the *C cell*. The C cell produces a hormone called *calcitonin*, which does not affect metabolism, but is involved in the regulation of calcium levels. This fact is useful because, after this cancer is treated by completely removing the thyroid, measurement of calcitonin levels at regular intervals is an easy way to diagnose a recurrence of this type of cancer. Medullary thyroid cancer is usually discovered when someone finds a lump. Other symptoms can include frequent loose stools and flushing of the skin.

Medullary thyroid cancer differs from the others in that it has a tendency to run in families. One out of every four people with medullary thyroid cancer has inherited the condition, which is linked with certain genes. If you inherit those genes, then you are almost certain to develop medullary thyroid cancer at some time. In hereditary cases, either another member of the family will also have medullary thyroid cancer or the person will have the medullary thyroid cancer as part of a condition called *multiple endocrine neoplasia (MEN)* syndrome in which cancer can occur in other glands, too.

Two different types of MEN exist. Patients with MEN type II-A have a tumour in an adrenal gland (called a *phaeochromocytoma*) and the parathyroid glands in the neck. The part of the adrenal gland affected (the middle bit, called the *medulla*) makes a hormone called *epinephrine* (also called adrenaline), which mimics the effects of stress in the body – so these people get high blood pressure. They also get elevated levels of calcium as a result of the parathyroid tumour. MEN type II-B also includes the adrenal tumour that produces excessive amounts of epinephrine, but not the parathyroid tumour. The third feature of MEN II-B is a characteristic physical appearance with tumours in the mouth.

In 75 per cent of occurrences, medullary thyroid cancer is not hereditary and no other family member has it, but family history is closely checked, just in case.

Even in the absence of symptoms suggesting other endocrine tumours, all people diagnosed with a medullary thyroid hormone are screened to exclude tumours of the adrenal and parathyroid glands. If present, controlling these tumours with medication before surgery is important, as high blood pressure makes surgery on your neck extremely dangerous.

The important characteristics of medullary thyroid cancer include:

- It's found in women more often than in men.

- It's not associated with exposure to radiation.

- It's more aggressive than papillary or follicular thyroid cancers, especially if it spreads to the lymph glands in the neck or to the bone and liver.

- If one family member is diagnosed with medullary thyroid cancer, other family members should have their calcitonin levels checked. If a family member's calcitonin is elevated, he or she should have the thyroid removed because cancer is almost always found or, if not yet present, will develop later.

- Even when the calcitonin is not elevated in a family member, genetic testing can determine whether that person may eventually get a medullary thyroid cancer (see Chapter 14).

- Measuring calcitonin levels reveals whether a tumour has spread or recurred after the removal of the thyroid.

Some thyroid specialists advocate measuring calcitonin as a screening test for all nodules suspected to contain thyroid cancer. So far, this practise is not routine as the diagnosis is readily made with a fine needle aspiration biopsy.

After 10 years, about 50 per cent of people with medullary thyroid cancer who receive treatment are still alive.

Undifferentiated (anaplastic) thyroid cancer

When thyroid cancer cells look so abnormal under a microscope that they do not resemble the thyroid cells from which they arose, the cells are described as *undifferentiated*. This type of cancer is very aggressive and rarely cured. While 95 per cent or more of people with a differentiated thyroid tumour, such as a papillary or follicular thyroid cancer, are alive and doing well after ten years, less than 10 per cent of those with undifferentiated thyroid cancer survive more than three years. Fortunately, undifferentiated cancer is rare, accounting for only about 2 per cent of all thyroid cancers.

This cancer is aggressive and invasive. While lymph node invasion in the case of papillary cancer is not a bad sign, lymph node invasion due to an undifferentiated cancer predicts a bad outcome.

The cancer tends to attach to local structures like nearby neck muscles, the trachea, the oesophagus, and blood vessels, making surgery very difficult, if not impossible. The outlook is so bad that there's little justification for extensive surgery that just causes mutilation without accomplishing a cure.

Important features of an undifferentiated cancer include:

- Males are affected twice as often as females.

- It usually occurs in people over the age of 65.

- It may occur in people with a distant history of radiation to the neck or face.

- At the time it's diagnosed, secondaries are often already found in local nodes and distant structures like the lungs, bone, brain, and liver.

- Most people will die of this type of cancer within six months to a year of diagnosis.

Staging Thyroid Cancer

For purposes of treatment, thyroid cancers are *staged* (divided into stages). This means they are divided into those stages where the cancer remains within the thyroid gland, those where the cancer has spread, and those according to the characteristics of the tumour, such as its size. Knowing which stage a cancer is in is important, because a follicular cancer that has the same stage as a papillary cancer responds to treatment in the same way, while two follicular cancers at very different stages respond differently.

Thyroid cancer is divided into four stages: I, II, III, and IV (see Table 8-1). Which stage of thyroid cancer a person has is based on the TNM classification, which stands for Tumour, Nodes, and Metastases (the posh word for secondaries, distant sites to which the cancer has spread via the bloodstream).

Using this classification, doctors describe whether the tumour (T) is less than or equal to 1 cm in greatest dimension (T1), between 1–4 cm in size (T2), greater than 4 cm in dimension (T3), whether it extends beyond the thyroid boundary capsule (T4, whatever its size), or is non-assessable (TX) because testing is not possible for some reason.

For the nodes (N), N0 means no nodes are involved, N1 means regional nodes are involved, while NX means the nodes are non-assessable. Similarly, for spread to other sites, M0 means no distant metastases, M1 means distant metastases, while MX means the presence of distant metastases is not assessable.

Someone whose tumour is diagnosed early is likely to have a TNM classification of: T1, N0, M0, meaning their primary tumour is less than 1 cm in dimension with no nodes or distant metastases involved, which is the essential basis for diagnosing a thyroid cancer as Stage I. The final staging does also depend on your age, and whether or not you are under or over 45 years.

Table 8-1	Papillary and Follicular Thyroid Cancer Staging	
	Under 45 Years	*45 Years and Older*
Stage I	Any T, any N, M0	T1, N0, M0
Stage II	Any T, any N, M1	T2, N0, M0
		T3, N0, M0
Stage III		T4, N0, M0
		Any T, N1, M0
Stage IV		Any T, any N, M1

So, for Stage I in someone under the age of 45 years, the key point for papillary and follicular cancers is that the tumour has not spread to distant sites, despite its size, and despite the involvement of local neck nodes. For someone over the age of 45 however, a Stage I cancer is only diagnosed if the tumour is less than 1 cm across (T1) and there are no nodes (N0) or metastases (M0). This diagnosis is made because age is an important factor in predicting the outcome of treatment in people with papillary and follicular thyroid cancers. If nodes are involved (N1) the cancer is always at least Stage III, whatever your age. If metastases are present, the cancer is always classed as Stage IV, whatever its size, node, or metastases status. Stage IV thyroid cancers usually contain undifferentiated cancer cells.

To make classification even more complex, the TNM basis for staging a medullary tumour is slightly different than for papillary and follicular cancers, as age is not a factor that predicts outcome for this type of tumour (see Table 8-2).

Table 8-2	Medullary Cancer Staging
Stage I	T1, N0, M0
Stage II	T2, N0, M0
	T3, N0, M0
	T4, N0, M0
Stage III	Any TI, N1, M0 (if nodes are involved, it's always at least Stage III)
Stage IV	Any T, any N, M1 (if metastases are present, it's always Stage IV)

If this information is starting to look too complicated for you to digest, don't worry – diagnosing the stage of your cancer is your doctor's job. Ask your doctor to explain it to you properly if you wish to know more.

Treating Thyroid Cancer

These guidelines suggest that someone with a suspected thyroid cancer should be urgently referred to a specialist thyroid clinic and seen within two weeks. At the clinic, the patient sees a multidisciplinary team made up of professionals who are interested in, and expert at, treating thyroid cancers. This team normally includes an endocrinologist, a surgeon, an oncologist (cancer specialist) with support from a pathologist, medical physicist, biochemist, radiologist, and specialist nurse. The guidelines also point out the importance of giving patients full verbal and written information about their condition and treatment, with continuing access to guidance and support as well as life-long follow-up.

The different types of thyroid cancer are treated in slightly different ways. If you have thyroid cancer your treatment usually starts as early as possible. In fact, national guidelines insist that all decisions relating to your diagnosis and treatment are made within two weeks of your first consultation, wherever possible. They also state that you receive an appointment to see the clinical oncologist (cancer specialist) or nuclear medicine physician (who is an expert in radioactive iodine treatment) within two weeks of referral from a surgeon. And, that after your surgery, arrangements for radioactive iodine treatment (if needed) are made within several weeks. In theory, that means that treatment is not subjected to unnecessary delays, which is good news.

Papillary thyroid cancer

Most people with papillary cancer, especially those with tumours greater than 1 cm in diameter, node involvement (N1), or secondaries (M1), and those with familial disease or disease due to radioactive exposure, undergo surgery to remove their entire thyroid gland (a total thyroidectomy) and local lymph nodes. The surgeon takes care to leave intact the tissue next to the parathyroid glands and recurrent laryngeal nerve. This procedure helps to ensure that the parathyroid glands continue to function and the person's speech is not damaged after surgery. If cancer is present in any lymph nodes, the surgeon removes as much non-essential tissue as possible, in what is known as a *modified radical neck dissection*.

In all cases, a total thyroidectomy is followed with radioactive iodine treatment to destroy any remaining thyroid tissue. After this, the person receives thyroxine hormone replacement at a dose that is high enough to suppress their natural production of thyroid stimulating hormone (TSH) from the pituitary gland (to less than 0.1 μU/ml (microunits per millilitre)). This dosage ensures that if a small remnant of thyroid tissue manages to survive both surgery and radioactive iodine treatment, TSH does not re-stimulate it into growth. Someone with a small papillary thyroid cancer of less than 1 cm in diameter and who has no nodes or metastases (T1, N0, M0) may undergo surgery to remove just the thyroid lobe in which the cancer is situated, plus the middle bit of the thyroid (isthmus). This operation is called a *lobectomy* and leaves part of the thyroid intact as the chance that cancer has spread into the other lobe is small. In this case, radioactive iodine is not given, and surgery is usually followed with thyroxine therapy to keep the TSH level suppressed.

Distant metastases develop in 5–20 per cent of patients with differentiated (papillary and follicular) thyroid cancers, mainly in the lungs and bones. Where they are accessible, surgical removal followed with radioactive iodine is the treatment of choice.

For secondaries in the bones, a combination of radioactive iodine, external beam radiotherapy, and orthopaedic surgery is used. For tumours that do not concentrate radioactive iodine, your management team will discuss other treatment options with you, such as *external beam radiotherapy* (in which the tumour is irradiated) and *chemotherapy* (using drugs that target rapidly dividing cancer cells) – both these approaches are designed to kill cancer cells so the tumour shrinks.

Follicular thyroid cancer

For follicular cancer, lobectomy is performed where the tumour is confined to the thyroid gland. If examination of the tumour under a microscope shows it's a type of follicular tumour known as a *follicular adenoma*, then no further treatment is needed. If the tumour is classed as a follicular cancer, however, and it is under 1 cm in diameter with no signs of invasion (T1, N0, M0), lobectomy is followed with thyroxine hormone replacement to suppress production of TSH.

If the follicular tumour is over 1 cm in diameter, fixed to surrounding tissues, or starting to invade local structures, then a total thyroidectomy is recommended, especially in older people, followed with radioactive iodine therapy and long-term suppression of TSH with thyroxine hormone replacement. Where the tumour has started to spread into local nodes, and where metastases are present, these are treated as for papillary cancer (see the previous section on treating papillary cancer).

Medullary thyroid cancer

As this type of tumour doesn't originate in thyroid-producing cells, its treatment is a little different. A surgeon removes the entire thyroid (total thyroidectomy) as well as dissecting out all the central neck nodes, as the fact that medullary cancer does not concentrate iodine means radioactive iodine does not eliminate thyroid tissue. The person's calcitonin level is measured at intervals to check for any regrowth of the tumour. External beam radiotherapy is sometimes used to control local recurrences, but is not used routinely as it doesn't improve survival rates. Similarly, chemotherapy is usually unhelpful, but is sometimes used if the disease is progressive.

Family members of someone with medullary thyroid cancer have their calcitonin levels checked regularly and, if their levels are high, will undergo investigation and treatment as well. Genetic testing is also available to rule out medullary thyroid cancer in other family members (see Chapter 14 for more on genetic testing).

Undifferentiated (anaplastic) thyroid cancer

This type of cancer is always classed as Stage IV as it's so aggressive and spreads so easily into surrounding tissues. Surgery is usually not considered as a good option, except when needed to maintain the airway if breathing is obstructed. Radioactive iodine therapy is not used either, as these immature cells do not concentrate iodine well. For this type of thyroid cancer, external beam radiotherapy is the mainstay of treatment, with or without chemotherapy.

Following Up Cancer Treatment

Anyone who has most or all of his or her thyroid gland removed starts taking thyroid hormone replacement after surgery and needs to continue that treatment for the rest of their life. Thyroid hormone replacement simply involves taking a daily pill of thyroxine hormone (refer to Chapter 5).

Someone treated for Stage I or II thyroid cancer usually has their blood levels of thyroglobulin (check out Chapter 3) checked regularly after surgery, too. If the level starts to rise, thyroid hormone replacement is stopped for several weeks. A full body scan with radioactive iodine is then carried out, looking for any evidence of thyroid tissue. If tissue is found, the person is given a much larger treatment dose of radioactive iodine to destroy the remaining thyroid tissue. The replacement thyroid hormone is then restarted a few days later.

Stopping the thyroid hormone allows the body to produce thyroid-stimulating hormone (TSH), which stimulates uptake of radioactive iodine within any remaining thyroid tissue. Instead of stopping thyroid hormone replacement, your doctor can give you synthetic TSH injections for several days prior to a thyroid scan with almost as good a result.

People with Stage III or IV thyroid cancer are likely to show regrowth of their tumour at some stage. This regrowth may respond to more external beam radiotherapy or to chemotherapy using chemicals known to destroy that type of tumour cell. Unfortunately, the outlook is poor for people with recurrent Stage III or IV thyroid cancer.

Chapter 9

Learning about Multinodular Goitres

Multinodular goitres – large thyroids with many nodules – are possibly the most common of all thyroid disorders. In various studies of people who died of other causes, between 30–60 per cent of them were found to have thyroid glands with multiple nodules. That means that up to 36 million people in the United Kingdom alone could have this disorder. What a workload for thyroid specialists! (With numbers like that, you wonder why nature placed the thyroid gland so prominently in the front of the neck near so many vital structures. Poor planning?)

Fortunately (or unfortunately, depending on which side of the desk you are sitting), most people with thyroid nodules never need treatment. Only a small fraction develop the signs and symptoms discussed in this chapter and need medical evaluation.

Exploring How a Multinodular Goitre Grows Up

Ryan (a distant cousin of our friend Kenneth from Chapter 7) is 46 years old. He goes to his doctor for a routine physical examination, and the doctor tells him that his thyroid feels bumpy. He has no symptoms in his neck. His doctor obtains thyroid function tests, which are normal, and thyroid autoantibody tests, which are negative. He is referred to the thyroid specialist clinic. (Check out Chapter 4 for more on thyroid autoantibodies and testing.)

The thyroid consultant examines Ryan and tells him that he can feel several distinct nodules, all of them soft and freely moveable. He sends Ryan for a thyroid scan, which shows that all the nodules can concentrate radioactive iodine (none of them are 'cold' – refer to Chapter 7). The consultant assures Ryan that he has a multinodular goitre and that no treatment is needed as long as he is free of symptoms. He asks Ryan to return in six months so that he can examine the thyroid again.

Four months later, Ryan suddenly feels pain in his neck and notices that one area has got larger. His doctor refers him back to the clinic, and the consultant inserts a needle in that area and removes a small amount of blood. He tells Ryan that a haemorrhage has occurred in one of the nodules, forming a cyst (a fluid-filled nodule) that requires no more treatment than evacuation of the blood. The pain occurs once more, and then it stops. Ryan returns every six months thereafter, and no further change takes place.

Ryan is an excellent illustration of the way that a multinodular goitre is typically discovered and evaluated and the most common outcome of the condition. Doctors believe that multinodular goitres result from some or all of the following circumstances:

✔ Starting around puberty, sometimes related to a deficiency of iodine (see Chapter 12), the thyroid is stimulated to grow. It grows a certain amount and then enters a resting state. This growth/resting cycle is repeated many times.

✔ The cells in the thyroid, though they almost all perform the same task of making thyroid hormone, are not identical and grow at different rates.

✔ Certain stresses to the body, such as pregnancy, increase the need for iodine, leading to more stimulation of the thyroid.

✔ Some foods called goitrogens (refer to Chapter 5) prevent the production of thyroid hormone and lead to more stimulation of the thyroid.

✔ Certain drugs, such as amiodarone (taken for heart rhythm irregularities), block production of thyroid hormone, which leads to more growth of the thyroid to compensate.

✔ A genetic connection may mean that multinodular goitres occur more often in some families than in others.

Figure 9-1 shows what a multinodular goitre looks like in comparison to a normal thyroid.

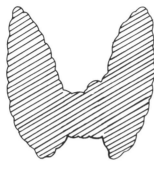 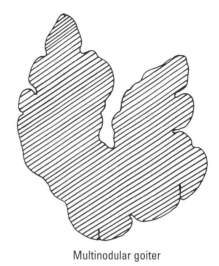

Figure 9-1:
A Multi-
nodular
goitre
compared
to a normal
thyroid.

Normal thyroid   Multinodular goiter

Ryan illustrates one way in which the goitre can be discovered, but goitres appear in many ways, including the following:

- A large neck suddenly gets much larger, leading to a visit to the doctor.

- Someone feels a sudden pain in his or her neck, and one side of his or her neck becomes larger because there's bleeding in a nodule.

- A doctor feels a large thyroid with many nodules during a routine examination.

- Symptoms develop such as a cough, difficulty swallowing, a feeling of pressure in the neck, or a lump in the throat.

- The goitre is discovered incidentally when other testing is carried out, like an ultrasound study of the neck or an X-ray of the chest.

- Occasionally, particularly in older people, the person develops a heart irregularity or signs and symptoms of hyperthyroidism (refer to Chapter 6 for more on hyperthyroidism).

Choosing to Treat It or Ignore It

Multinodular goitres generally proceed along the same path in most people. When thyroid function tests are done, the results are either normal or the thyroid hormone levels are elevated, suggesting hyperthyroidism; the thyroid hormone levels are rarely low. If someone experiences sudden pain in one area of the thyroid, the thyroid specialist performs a fine needle aspiration biopsy (check out Chapter 4). Usually that area of the thyroid contains blood as a result of a haemorrhage in one of the nodules. When the blood is removed, the nodule shrinks.

If a particular nodule stands out or is harder than the others, the nodule is (Q:?biopsied) and is usually diagnosed as benign. If the nodule is cancerous, treatment for cancer is begun (refer to Chapter 8).

If the only problem is the large gland, most of the time the doctor doesn't treat it. If the person experiences other symptoms in the neck or if the thyroid gland is particularly unsightly, treatment is usually offered.

Sometimes the thyroid, instead of growing up and out, grows downward behind the breastbone (the sternum) and is described as *substernal*. In this position, where there is little room to grow, the thyroid can squeeze other organs like the *trachea* (the air pipe from the throat to the lungs). Treatment is then necessary to reduce symptoms that arise from this condition.

Most people with a multinodular goitre don't realise they have it, and even if they're aware that it exists, they don't find treating it necessary.

Making a Diagnosis

Depending upon how a multinodular goitre is discovered, a doctor can do a number of studies to determine exactly what's going on in the thyroid gland.

A good pair of expert hands can feel the presence of many nodules (although no one can feel nodules smaller than one centimetre in size). This examination is very important because it serves as a baseline for future thyroid exams. The doctor notes the size of the thyroid so she can compare what she feels during future examinations to determine if the thyroid is growing.

The first study of a multinodular goitre consists of thyroid function tests to see whether the thyroid is making the right amount of thyroid hormone. These test results are usually normal, but occasionally they show excess production of thyroid hormone. Thyroid autoantibody tests are sometimes requested, especially if the person has a family history of goitres. These test results are usually negative unless autoimmune thyroiditis is present (refer to Chapter 5).

If thyroid function tests indicate hyperthyroidism, the doctor looks for other signs of hyperthyroidism due to Graves' disease. Thyroid eye and skin disease, described in Chapter 6, supports a diagnosis of Graves' disease. A patient who has hyperthyroidism in a multinodular goitre has a condition called *toxic multinodular goitre*, also known as *Plummer's disease*.

When one nodule stands out or is harder than the others, the doctor does a fine needle aspiration biopsy to rule out cancer. A thyroid scan may precede the biopsy to see whether the nodule is functional (warm or hot) or if it's cold (refer to Chapter 7). Cancers are usually cold. However, keep in mind that the majority of cold nodules are not cancer. If cancer isn't present, the fine needle biopsy doesn't add any information that points to a diagnosis of the multinodular goitre.

A thyroid scan gives a general picture of the thyroid, showing the size of the gland, the many nodules, and the position of the gland, which is particularly important if it has grown down below the sternum (see the previous section, 'Choosing to Treat It or Ignore It').

A thyroid ultrasound test picks up very small nodules. This test is used to show whether a tender nodule is a cyst – a fluid-filled nodule – or solid.

If someone feels significant pressure in their neck or has trouble swallowing, the doctor may arrange a barium swallow: The person swallows barium, and X-rays are taken as it passes down the throat. This test may show that the thyroid gland is putting pressure on the oesophagus, the swallowing tube from the mouth to the stomach. A plain film (without barium) of the neck reveals if the trachea is deviated by the mass of the thyroid.

Thyroid function tests are always done when someone has a multinodular goitre. Depending on the stress the person feels from this growth in the neck and on how important the doctor thinks it is to leave no stone unturned, many, all, or none of the other tests described in this section are carried out.

Treating a Multinodular Goitre

If the nodules of a multinodular goitre aren't causing symptoms of hyperthyroidism and don't contain cancer, and if the person has no symptoms, the multinodular goitre is usually left alone.

Doctors used to think they could shrink a multinodular goitre with thyroid hormone, but this is not the case.

If the person dislikes the appearance of his or her neck, or if they are hyperthyroid, radioactive iodine is used to destroy some of the thyroid tissue (see Chapter 6). This treatment works even for large goitres but sometimes results in hypothyroidism. Also, in the course of destroying thyroid tissue, a lot of thyroid hormone is released into the blood stream, inducing temporary hyperthyroidism if it isn't present already. Older people, especially, need to receive antithyroid drugs before using radioactive iodine (see Chapter 6).

Some people (less than 10 per cent) who are given radioactive iodine to shrink a large multinodular goitre, develop Graves' disease, which is discussed in Chapter 6. This complication happens because tissue is released into the blood stream, and the body forms antibodies against it.

Surgery is very rarely carried out for a multinodular goitre unless a cancer is found. Radioactive iodine is able to treat most of these thyroid glands, even the large ones that grow in a downward direction (substernal). If surgery is needed for a benign multinodular goitre, enough thyroid tissue is left to keep the patient functionally normal. Thyroid hormone pills are not given unless hypothyroidism develops subsequently. Even if they were given straightaway, they wouldn't prevent such a gland from growing again.

Patients with multinodular goitres should return to their doctors at least annually to have an examination of the thyroid, or earlier when new growth is seen or pain develops.

Part III
Managing Your Thyroid

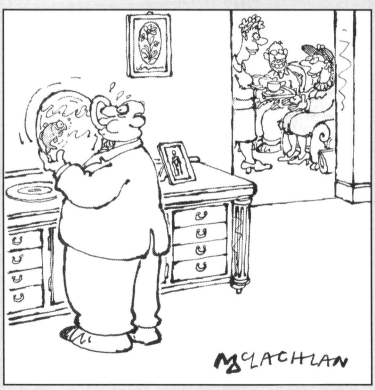

"They guessed Neville had a thyroid problem because of his excessive thirst, so they put him on a high fish diet."

In this part . . .

*T*hese chapters clue you into some special situations that can affect your thyroid, particularly infections and medications you take for other conditions. We explain the most prevalent thyroid disorder, iodine deficiency disease. If you must have thyroid surgery, we tell you what to expect and how to prepare.

Plus, there is plenty you can do to keep your thyroid happy and making those essential hormones in the right quantities. In this part we discuss some ways you can manage your body so that thyroid function takes place in a healthy environment, and give you the low-down on alternative therapies.

Chapter 10

Taking Care with Drugs That Affect Your Thyroid

As thyroid hormones affect every cell in your body, you won't be surprised to hear that lots of drugs have an effect on your thyroid function as an unwanted side effect. Certain chemicals in your food and in the environment can change thyroid function, too. Whether you have high blood pressure, a headache, or heart failure, at some point you're bound to run into drugs that affect your thyroid function in some way. You need to know about these side effects so that changes in your thyroid hormone levels or your metabolism that result from one of them, doesn't lead to wrong conclusions about the state of your thyroid health.

In this chapter, you meet most of the important drugs that interact with your thyroid in one way or another.

Revealing the Drug–Food–Thyroid Connection

Natasha is a 36-year-old woman who's healthy and wants to avoid having any more children, as her family is complete. She asks her doctor for the oral contraceptive pill. One day, while browsing in a bookstore, she comes upon *Thyroid For Dummies*, by Alan Rubin and Sarah Brewer (Wiley). (She can't miss it; it's featured in the 'Must Read' section of the bookshop.) She opens it and reads on the Cheat Sheet at the front of the book that thyroid problems can run in families. As several of her relatives have an overactive thyroid gland, she returns to her doctor to ask if getting a thyroid function test would be a good idea.

Her doctor, unfortunately, is away, and the inexperienced locum, who has not read the book, still tests thyroid function with a total thyroxine test (refer to Chapter 4). The result is high. He tells Natasha that she may have hyper-thyroidism. Natasha reads further in the book and finds that the oestrogen in her oral contraceptive pill raises the amount of thyroid-binding protein in her system. Meanwhile, the free thyroxine, the form of the thyroid hormone that can enter cells and, therefore, have an effect, remains normal. She informs the (embarrassed) locum, who does a free T4 test and a TSH (thyroid-stimulating hormone) test, both of which are normal. No further treatment is needed.

Leonard is a 72-year-old man who is having trouble with a very irregular heartbeat. His doctor places him on a drug to correct irregular heartbeats called amiodarone. About two months later, Leonard's heartbeat is regular, but he is beginning to feel cold and sleepy. He has gained a few pounds and notices that his skin is dry. His doctor recognises the symptoms of hypothy-roidism (check out Chapter 5), sometimes associated with amiodarone. The doctor orders thyroid function tests to confirm the diagnosis and starts Leonard on thyroid hormone. In a month, he has returned to his normal state of health.

Kathy has seen her doctor for many years because of a multinodular goitre, which has needed no treatment until now. At the age of 68, she develops a rapid heartbeat and sees a cardiologist. She is placed on amiodarone (the same medication that Leonard takes), and her heart problem resolves. However, after six weeks, she notices that her heart is beating rapidly again. Not only that, she is losing weight and having trouble sleeping. She feels warm all the time although she is well past her menopause.

Kathy returns to the cardiologist, who recognises that her symptoms are a side effect of amiodarone and refers her to the local thyroid specialist clinic. Here, the consultant tells Kathy that she has hyperthyroidism due to the effect of amiodarone on her multinodular goitre. He suggests that she takes a drug to control the thyroid and stop taking the amiodarone if the cardiologist can substitute another drug.

Kathy is able to stop the amiodarone and takes a drug called carbimazole, but her condition does not improve. After two months, the thyroid consultant rec-ommends surgery. After the thyroid surgery is performed, Kathy improves dra-matically. She is now able to take the amiodarone and feels fine.

George absolutely loves broccoli and consumes prodigious quantities, even at breakfast. He finds that he is often sleepy and cold. He has trouble thinking and making appropriate decisions. He goes to his doctor, who requests blood tests that show a high thyroid stimulating hormone (TSH). The doctor tells George that he is hypothyroid and puts him on thyroid medication.

One night, George and his wife invite Natasha and her husband to dinner. As Natasha watches George consume huge quantities of broccoli, she remarks that she has read in *Thyroid for Dummies* that broccoli contains a substance that reduces thyroid function. George is very surprised to hear this news, but he sharply reduces his broccoli intake after that night. After talking over the situation with his doctor, he also gradually reduces his thyroid hormone replacement. After he's been off the broccoli for a month, George's thyroid tests are normal.

How drugs affect your thyroid hormones

Chapter 3 explains how thyroid hormones are made and released, how they are carried around the body, how they are taken up by cells where they do their work, and how they work within these cells. Drugs can affect thyroid function at any one or more of these levels.

Thyroid hormone is formed when iodine is added to a compound called thyronine. When four iodine molecules are attached to this compound, the result is thyroxine (T4). When three molecules of iodine are attached, the compound produced is triiodothyronine (T3). T3 is also produced by removing one iodine molecule from thyroxine. Many drugs and food substances block the production of both T4 and T3.

After T3 and T4 are produced, they must travel in the body to get to their site of action. They are carried in the blood stream by thyroid-binding proteins (refer to Chapter 3). Drugs can affect thyroid function by increasing or decreasing the amount of binding protein in the blood. In this case, thyroid test results are affected even though thyroid function remains normal. This result occurs because it's the free thyroid hormone (hormone not bound to protein) that is active in the body, not the hormone that's attached to protein.

The free hormone arrives at the cell where it needs to do its work, and gets into the cell by attaching to a special receptor on the cell membrane. The receptor is yet another place where certain drugs can prevent thyroid hormone from doing its job, for example, if they block the receptors so no hormone can enter. The situation is almost like diabetes, in which plenty of glucose (sugar) is available in the blood stream for energy, but it can't enter the cell where it does its work.

Once inside the cell, thyroid hormone attaches to the nucleus, where the genetic material is stored. The hormone then encourages a certain action to take place within that cell. Various drugs can block the hormone's attachment to the nucleus or alter the attachment so that it doesn't produce the desired effect.

These cases illustrate the broad spectrum of effects that various drugs and foods can have on thyroid function. Some drugs affect thyroid function tests while the thyroid itself is still normal. Other drugs can create hypothyroidism or hyperthyroidism. As if these effects aren't confusing enough, the same drug given to two different people may cause opposite effects, depending on their particular clinical situation.

This chapter describes the main drugs that affect thyroid function or thyroid function tests. At the end of this chapter, these drugs are grouped according to their main clinical purpose so that you can check if any drug you're taking – for example, to treat high blood pressure, diabetes, or fluid retention – could affect you. As drugs are mainly described using their generic (non-trademarked) name in the United Kingdom, these generic names are the ones used here. If you are not certain whether the drug you are taking is likely to affect your thyroid, you can always ask your pharmacist; your pharmacist is probably more of an expert on the way that drugs work, and their possible side effects, than your doctor.

New medicines are coming on to the market almost every day. Although these products get better and better at curing diseases, their other effects are often not known from the few thousand people who test them before they come to market. The side effects of many drugs don't become clear until hundreds of thousands of people have taken them. Many, if not all, of these new drugs affect the thyroid in one way or another. The people who must pay particular attention are those who have some underlying thyroid disease to begin with. For example:

✔ If you've had hyperthyroidism (refer to Chapter 6) and it's under control with antithyroid drugs, a drug containing a lot of iodine will probably cause a recurrence of your disease.

✔ If you've had a multinodular goitre (refer to Chapter 9), iodine will possibly bring on hyperthyroidism.

✔ If you're borderline hypothyroid (refer to Chapter 5), iodine or one of the drugs that block thyroid hormone production will bring on clinical hypothyroidism.

✔ If you have mild subacute thyroiditis (head to Chapter 11), some drugs will make it worse to the point that you experience symptoms.

Identifying the Effects of Specific Substances

In this section, you encounter particular drugs that affect the thyroid, grouped together according to their potential impact on your thyroid.

Initiating or aggravating hypothyroidism

Many drugs have the potential to cause or intensify hypothyroidism. The parts of this section look at the most commonly prescribed medications to have this potential side effect.

Drugs that compete with iodine

If iodine can't enter your thyroid, you can't make thyroid hormone, and you experience hypothyroidism. Some drugs compete with iodine for entry into the thyroid. Usually the effect is mild, and hypothyroidism doesn't occur. But if your diet is limited in iodine, these drugs can cause low thyroid function.

The most important drug in this category is lithium, which is used to treat manic-depression. In one study, as many as 10 per cent of people given lithium became hypothyroid. This effect is much more common in women than in men and occurs within the first two years of treatment. Most likely, the large population of women with autoimmune thyroid disease (refer to Chapter 5) is most susceptible to the antithyroid effect of lithium. Not only does lithium block the uptake of iodine, but it also inhibits the production and release of thyroid hormone. Some people taking lithium develop a goitre. Curiously (and rarely), lithium can cause hyperthyroidism rather than hypothyroidism.

The mineral fluorine, which is found mainly in fluoridised water and dental products, has a similar effect on the thyroid. If you consume substantial amounts of fluorine, your thyroid will decrease its production of T4. Your pituitary gland then makes more TSH to stimulate the thyroid, and you can end up with a goitre.

Drugs that prevent the addition of iodine to form thyroid hormones

Another group of medications blocks the production of thyroid hormones in a slightly different way. These medications keep iodine from combining with thyronine to form either T4 or T3, the two thyroid hormones. This group of medications includes:

- **Aminoglutethimide:** Used in the treatment of breast and prostate cancer, although it's now largely replaced with newer, better tolerated drugs. As many as one-third of patients treated with this medication develop hypothyroidism.

- **Ketoconazole:** Used as an antifungal drug. Hypothyroidism is a rare side effect of this agent.

- **Sulfonamide drugs:** Used to eliminate excess water from the body and act as antibiotics, such as sulfadiazine and acetazolamide. If you use these diuretics and antibiotics for prolonged periods of time, they can cause hypothyroidism.

✓ **Sulphonylureas:** Used in the treatment of diabetes, such as tolbutamide and chlorpropamide.

✓ **Antithyroid drugs:** Used to treat hypothyroidism, such as propylth-iouracil and carbimazole

Two chemicals found in food have an impact similar to the medications in the preceding list to produce hypothyroidism. They are

✓ **Isoflavones:** Found in soybeans. Children fed on large amounts of soy products may develop a goitre.

✓ **Thiocyanate:** Contained in many vegetables, such as:

- Broccoli

- Brussels sprouts

- Cauliflower

- Cabbage

- Horseradish

- Kale

- Kohlrabi

- Mustard

- Swede

- Turnips

If cattle consume foods like these and you drink milk from those cattle, your thyroid is sometimes affected as well.

Drugs that affect the transport of thyroid hormone

Many drugs affect how thyroid hormones are transported in your bloodstream. Chances are you'll take one of these drugs at some point in your life. If you have normal thyroid function, your thyroid simply makes more or less thyroid hormone to compensate for the effects of these drugs. However, if you're hypothyroid and taking a thyroid hormone replacement, you may need to adjust your dose when taking one of these drugs.

The following drugs increase thyroid-binding protein, resulting in an increase in total (but not free) thyroxine unless you get your thyroid hormone as a medication:

✔ **Oestrogens:** The most commonly used drugs in this category. For years, oestrogens caused confusion with respect to thyroid function because doctors used to measure how much total thyroxine was in your system, not just how much free thyroxine is there (refer to Chapter 4). Oestrogens are found in the combined oral contraceptive pill and hormone replacement therapy. Some animals are fed oestrogens to fatten them up, so as you consume those animals, you get oestrogen that way as well. The list of medications that contain oestrogens is huge.

✔ **Clofibrate:** A drug used for lowering blood fats.

✔ **Perphenazine:** A treatment for psychotic disorders in the group of drugs called phenothiazines. This group includes a number of well-known medications, such as prochlorperazine, trifluoperazine, and chlorpromazine. Perphenazine is the main ingredient in a number of different preparations and is also used for treating nausea and vomiting.

The following drugs decrease thyroid-binding protein resulting in a decrease in total (but not free) thyroxine unless you get your thyroid hormone as a medication:

✔ **Androgens:** A substitute for the male hormone, testosterone, when a man cannot make his own. They permit muscle growth and normal sexual function.

✔ **Corticosteroids:** Used extensively to treat inflammation and to reduce immunity when inflammation and autoimmunity are damaging the body, such as in rheumatoid arthritis and many other illnesses. The list of corticosteroids is a long one.

✔ **Nicotinic acid:** A vitamin used for the treatment of elevated fats in the blood.

If you are hypothyroid and are put on one of these agents for a long time, ensure that your doctor remembers to check your thyroid function periodically.

The opiates heroin and methadone also affect the movement of thyroid hormones in the blood stream.

Amiodarone

Amiodarone is used for disturbances of the heart rhythm. This drug may cause hypothyroidism in up to 10 per cent of the people who take it. The drug is also associated with a number of other side effects, including skin and corneal discolouration and fibrosis of the lungs. It may cause hepatitis and bone marrow suppression. Despite all these negatives, the drug is very useful in treating heart rhythm disturbances.

Drugs used to treat severe hyperthyroidism

The drugs in this group are useful when an individual has severe hyperthyroidism and needs to reduce the T3 hormone level as soon as possible. However, these drugs have other primary purposes, and when they are prescribed for those other purposes (to patients who aren't hyperthyroid), they can create hypothyroidism.

- ✔ **Corticosteroids:** These drugs are discussed in the previous section.

- ✔ **Iodinated contrast agents:** These drugs are used for achieving better X-ray studies. A single dose can last for 10 days.

- ✔ **Propranolol:** Used to slow a rapid heartbeat, but it's also used to treat hyperthyroidism because it controls many of the symptoms, such as palpitations, shakiness, and nervousness.

- ✔ **Propylthiouracil:** One of the standard drugs for the treatment of hyperthyroidism in the United Kingdom.

Growth hormone

When the body does not make its own growth hormone, an injectable growth hormone restores growth. Growth hormone is administered to children who are not growing properly because they lack this hormone. If someone is borderline hypothyroid, this hormone may push him into hypothyroidism as it reduces the T4 hormone to abnormally low levels.

Drugs that remove thyroid hormone from your system

A number of drugs act upon the liver to speed up the metabolism of thyroid hormones into products that are not active. Other drugs pull thyroid hormones out of the body with bowel movements. These drugs are very common.

If you are taking a thyroid replacement hormone and you use one of these drugs, you may develop hypothyroidism. Ask your doctor to check your thyroid hormone levels about a month after you start taking one of these drugs:

- ✔ **Aluminium hydroxide:** Used to treat peptic ulcers.

- ✔ **Carbamazepine and phenytoin:** Used to treat convulsions.

- ✔ **Colestyramine and colestipol:** Used to reduce fats.

- ✔ **Ferrous sulphate:** Given to people who are deficient in iron and have anaemia. At some point, the ferrous sulphate treatment is stopped when the person's iron reserves are full. The person may actually become hyperthyroid at that point, if his thyroid hormone dose was increased due to the initial effects of the drug.

- ✔ **Phenobarbital:** Used for the treatment of convulsions.

✔ **Rifampicin:** One of the treatments for tuberculosis. This drug very rarely causes hypothyroidism in a person who takes thyroid hormone.

✔ **Sucralfate:** Used for peptic ulcer disease. It may result in hypothyroidism if it's taken long-term.

Importantly, you need to monitor your thyroid function both during and after use of a short-term medication that lowers the levels of thyroid hormone in your blood, especially if you are taking oral thyroid medication.

Drugs that decrease your TSH

The following drugs can lower the level of thyroid-stimulating hormone in your system, potentially leading to lower thyroid function:

✔ **Acetylsalicylic acid:** This drug is more commonly known as aspirin. People taking more than 8 or 10 aspirin daily may suffer this effect on TSH.

✔ **Bromocriptine:** Given to prevent lactation (milk production) and to shrink prolactin-secreting pituitary tumours.

✔ **Dopamine:** Used to lower blood pressure, especially in an emergency setting. It lowers TSH but is not usually used long enough to cause problems with hypothyroidism.

✔ **Corticosteroids:** Used to treat inflammation and reduce immunity.

✔ **Octreotide:** A drug that treats certain tumours that produce hormones, especially acromegaly, which produces excessive growth hormone, and carcinoid tumours, which produce a chemical that causes severe diarrhoea and flushing of the skin.

✔ **Opiates:** Drugs including morphine and heroin (diamorphine), which are used legally for pain control and illegally for a chemical high.

✔ **Phentolamine:** Given to control blood pressure in someone with a tumour of the adrenal gland called a phaeochromocytoma. It reduces TSH but is not generally given long enough to make a difference in thyroid function.

✔ **Pyridoxine:** Also called vitamin B6. This drug is taken for premenstrual syndrome, and when a person shows evidence of B6 vitamin deficiency.

✔ **Thyroid hormones:** Given to replace a deficiency or to suppress thyroid cancer or a goitre. They suppress the production of TSH.

Creating false test results

Certain drugs can alter the thyroid hormone (T3 and T4) tests that measure total thyroid hormones (but not free thyroid hormones, which remain normal).

If you're taking one of the drugs listed here, keep that fact in mind if your total T4 test shows hypothyroidism but you aren't experiencing any symptoms of the condition.

- **Salicylates:** Aspirin is the most commonly used drug in this group.

- **Phenytoin and carbamazepine:** Used as treatment for convulsions.

- **Furosemide:** Causes the loss of excess water through the kidneys.

- **Heparin:** Used to prevent blood clots. This drug doesn't change your thyroid function, but if you're given an injection of low molecular weight heparin, a measurement of free T4 taken within 10 hours of the injection is falsely elevated.

- **Orphenadrine:** Used in a number of drug preparations for the relief of muscle spasms. It is not a muscle relaxant but may reduce pain.

Causing an increase in thyroid activity

The following drugs increase the production of TSH, which can result in hyperthyroidism:

- **Amphetamine:** A controlled drug sometimes used inappropriately as a weight-loss agent.

- **Cimetidine and ranitidine:** Used to reduce acid secretion to treat peptic ulcers. Both can raise the TSH, but studies don't show a change in thyroid function with these drugs.

- **Clomifene:** Brings on ovulation to promote pregnancy. It has effects on several of the hormones in the pituitary gland, including TSH.

- **L-dopa inhibitors:** Drugs such as chlorpromazine and haloperidol, used in the management of psychotic disorders. They raise TSH, although people do not generally become hyperthyroid.

- **Metoclopramide and domperidone:** Used to control nausea and vomiting, especially after surgery.

- **Iodine:** Raises TSH levels as it blocks the release of thyroid hormones.

- **Lithium:** Raises TSH, in addition to all its other effects on thyroid function. In very rare cases, it can cause hyperthyroidism. (It causes hypothyroidism much more frequently.)

Preventing Harmful Drug Interactions

With so many drugs having an effect on thyroid function in one way or another, avoiding drug interactions becomes very difficult, particularly if one of the drugs you're taking is thyroid hormone. If you're taking thyroid hormone, your body isn't able to make the subtle changes in thyroid function necessary to compensate for the other drug you're taking, which is most likely reducing the thyroid hormone available to your systems. The best solution is to ask your pharmacist to check for interactions between the drugs you are taking, and your thyroid function.

Discovering Whether You're at Risk

The drugs named in this chapter are given as their generic names. The generic name is the official name of the drug regardless of the name the manufacturer gives it, as all general practitioners (GPs) are encouraged to prescribe drugs generically for cost purposes.

This section groups the drugs according to their usage. If you have a specific medical problem – for example, diabetes – go to that section, look at the drugs listed there, and see whether the generic drug is the same as the one you're using.

If one of the drugs listed here is something you take, ask your doctor if you need a thyroid function test:

- ✔ Anaemia drugs, such as ferrous sulphate

- ✔ Anti-addiction agents, such as methadone

- ✔ Antibiotics, including:

    - Ketoconazole

    - Sulfonamide drugs: co-trimoxazole, sulfadiazine

    - Rifampicin

- ✔ Anti-inflammatory drugs, such as:

    - Corticosteroid tablets: prednisolone, betamethasone, cortisone acetate, deflazacort, dexamethasone, hydrocortisone, methyl-prednisolone

    - Aspirin

✔ Antithyroid drugs:

- Propylthiouracil

- Carbimazole

✔ Drugs that suppress growth hormone, such as octreotide

✔ Nausea control drugs, such as:

- Domperidone

- Metoclopramide

- Prolactin control drugs, such as Bromocriptine

✔ Diabetes drugs, including:

- Tolbutamide

- Chlorpropamide

✔ Diuretics (drugs that reduce body water):

- Furosemide

✔ Fat-lowering drugs:

- Colestyramine

- Colestipol

✔ Heart rhythm drugs:

- Amiodarone

- Propranolol

- Phentolamine

✔ Hormone replacements:

- Oestrogens (female hormones): found in the combined oral contraceptive pill, and in hormone replacement therapy

- Androgens (male hormones): testosterone

- Growth hormone

- Clomiphene

- Thyroid hormones: thyroxine sodium (T4), levothyroxine sodium (T4), liothyronine sodium (T3)

✔ Pain medication:

- Morphine

- Diamorphine

✔ Peptic ulcer drugs:

- Aluminium hydroxide
- Sucralfate
- Cimetidine
- Ranitidine

✔ Psychoactive drugs:

- Lithium
- Perphenazine
- Chlorpromazine
- Haloperidol

.

Chapter 11

Spotting Thyroid Infections and Inflammation

*T*he term *thyroiditis* is used in this book (check out Chapter 5) to mean the most common form of apparent inflammation of the thyroid, autoimmune thyroiditis – also known as Hashimoto's thyroiditis and chronic thyroiditis. This chapter also introduces you to causes of thyroiditis that are less common than autoimmune disorders but just as important to know about. Usually, but not always, thyroiditis is associated with infection.

Fortunately, infection of the thyroid is rare, perhaps because of all the anti-septic iodine and hydrogen peroxide found within the thyroid gland. Despite all this natural protection, every so often people develop an infected thyroid. In this chapter, you discover how doctors tell one form of infection from another, as well as the method of treatment and the prognosis for each illness.

Putting a Face on Subacute Thyroiditis

Joan is a 40-year-old woman who is suffering from a cough and cold with a low-grade fever for more than a week. One morning, she wakes to notice that her neck hurts. She can tell that the pain is located in the centre of her neck beneath her Adam's apple. She goes to her doctor, who notes that her thyroid is enlarged and tender. The doctor also finds that Joan is nervous, and her fingers are shaking slightly.

Her GP sends Joan for a thyroid function test, which shows that her free T4 is elevated while her TSH is depressed (refer to Chapter 4), suggesting hyperthyroidism. The doctor also requests a test for inflammation called an *erythrocyte sedimentation rate (ESR)* and the result is elevated. Knowing that neck pain is unusual in hyperthyroidism due to Grave's disease (find out more in Chapter 6), the GP phones the thyroid specialist clinic who has a free appointment to see Joan the next day.

At the clinic, blood is taken to measure Joan's serum thyroglobulin level, which comes back high, while the uptake of radioactive iodine is low (refer to Chapter 4). Joan finds out that she has subacute thyroiditis. She is started on aspirin and rapidly improves. The swelling of her neck declines, and the tenderness rapidly decreases.

Causes and effects

Subacute thyroiditis has many names including De Quervain's thyroiditis, giant cell thyroiditis, and subacute painful thyroiditis. The condition is called *subacute* to differentiate it from a similar condition, *acute thyroiditis*, which is usually much more painful and associated with more symptoms that make the person sick.

Subacute thyroiditis is not very common, and typically accounts for less than 10 per cent of all cases of thyrotoxicosis.

As you see from Joan's case, this condition often begins with an infection that suggests a virus. The person may have muscle aches and fever, and then begins to feel neck pain in the area of the thyroid. This pain is sometimes severe and usually brings the person to their doctor. When the doctor examines the patient, the thyroid is not only painful but enlarged as well.

Evidence exists that subacute thyroiditis is due to a virus: Cases of this condition are often seasonal, and they sometimes occur in outbreaks like any infectious disease. Over the years, doctors looking for a particular virus that might cause all cases of subacute thyroiditis have had little luck. The only virus that is found with some frequency is the mumps virus.

Subacute thyroiditis seems to occur more often in people with low immunity from an infection, such as AIDS (acquired immune deficiency syndrome), or people who receive bone marrow transplants for leukaemia.

As a result of the inflammation, the thyroid releases much of its stored hormone along with the stored thyroglobulin (refer to Chapter 4), resulting in hyperthyroidism. The virus also seems to temporarily damage thyroid cells and, as production of thyroid hormone isn't ongoing, the hyperthyroidism lasts only a brief time, sometimes only a few days, until the thyroid gland is depleted of hormone. The person then goes through a brief period of normal thyroid function as hormone levels fall, before swinging into the opposite condition, hypothyroidism. Finally, because a viral illness usually doesn't last, the thyroid gland returns to normal, the pain goes away, and the thyroid function returns to normal.

Like most thyroid conditions, subacute thyroiditis is more common in women than men; the ratio of cases is 3 to 1. This condition appears to have some genetic basis because the same genetic marker – an antigen on human white blood cells – is found in about 75 per cent of cases, suggesting that people who inherit this marker are more susceptible to the disease. In fact, two different genetic markers have been described. Interestingly, each one is associated with the disease occurring at a different time of the year, although in either case it generally occurs in the fourth or fifth decade of life.

A small (about 2 per cent) but definite possibility of a recurrence is likely some years later. This recurrence is generally milder than the original attack, although occasionally, someone may experience repeated attacks of pain. Thyroid hormone helps to prevent such recurrences, but if recurrences keep coming back, removing the thyroid with surgery or radioactive iodine is necessary.

Laboratory findings

Lab tests are very helpful in pinning down a diagnosis of subacute thyroiditis. Some of the findings are as follows:

- The erythrocyte sedimentation rate (ESR), a general blood test for inflammation, is often unusually high considering the relative mildness of the symptoms.

- Shortly after the thyroid becomes infected, up to 50 per cent of people experience hyperthyroidism, so TSH levels are low while FT4 levels are elevated.

- Inflammation causes the release of a large quantity of both T4 and T3. Because the thyroid contains so much more T4 relative to T3, compared to the blood, a drop in the ratio of T4 to T3 is experienced as they escape into the blood stream.

- If liver tests are done, the level of alkaline phosphatase is often elevated. It appears that the infection affects the liver in addition to the thyroid, though the impact on the liver is mild.

✔ Blood tests show that a lot of thyroglobulin is present in the blood.

✔ The test for thyroid autoantibodies (refer to Chapter 4) is negative.

✔ Some specialists suggest that a thyroid ultrasound study (refer to Chapter 4) is distinctive in subacute thyroiditis, but this test is not usually done.

✔ The key test, the thyroid uptake of radioactive iodine, is very low, which differentiates this condition from other causes of hyperthyroidism.

When the results of all these tests and the clinical picture are put together, the diagnosis is fairly certain; although no one test proves that subacute thyroiditis is present. To prove the diagnosis, a biopsy of the gland is necessary, but the mildness of the disease means that a biopsy is rarely done.

Subacute thyroiditis differs from other forms of thyroiditis as it causes generalised thyroid pain, though sometimes the pain occurs on one side of the thyroid only. Another cause of a painful thyroid is bleeding, producing a haemorrhagic thyroid cyst. This pain usually occurs on one side of the thyroid and is not associated with a viral illness. Lab tests help to secure a diagnosis, particularly a radioactive uptake, which is normal for the cystic thyroid but low for subacute thyroiditis. In rare cases, chronic thyroiditis is painful (refer to Chapter 5). With chronic thyroiditis, levels of thyroid auto-antibodies are high.

Treatment options

At the beginning of subacute thyroiditis, when someone is hyperthyroid, a drug such as propranolol is sometimes used to reverse the symptoms of excessive thyroid hormone. (Propranolol is a beta-blocker that slows the heart, decreases anxiety, and reduces tremor.) Antithyroid drugs like propylthiouracil and carbimazole have no place in this treatment, because the thyroid is not making excessive hormones long-term.

Often, the only treatment needed is aspirin or a non-steroidal anti-inflammatory agent, such as ibuprofen. Once in a while, using a corticosteroid, such as prednisolone, is necessary for a week or two. When the uptake of radioactive iodine returns to normal, the inflammation is finished, and any corticosteroids are stopped.

With the end of symptoms, the patient is back to normal permanently in almost every case. Like so much in medicine, rare exceptions do arise where the disease goes away and then returns or the pain is persistent. In these rare cases, removing the thyroid may prove necessary to finally control the disease.

Coping with Postpartum and Silent Thyroiditis

Michelle is a 29-year-old woman who has a healthy 5-month-old baby boy. She notices that her neck is larger than before, but it's not painful. She is feeling nervous, her hands shake, and she feels her heart beating rapidly at times. She has trouble going to sleep, which makes her situation tough because the baby often wakes her up at night, too.

Michelle sees her family doctor, who examines her and tells her that she is probably hyperthyroid. The doctor notes that Michelle was pregnant recently and requests thyroid function tests, which are elevated. After referral to the thyroid specialist clinic, Michelle finds out that she probably has postpartum thyroiditis. The consultant places her on the beta-blocker called propranolol, which controls her symptoms well. The consultant also explains that she will probably go through a phase of low thyroid function before returning to normal.

Several weeks after seeing the consultant, Michelle notices that she's feeling cold and having trouble keeping awake. Her GP reassures her that experiencing these symptoms is the hypothyroid phase of postpartum thyroiditis and, within a few weeks, she feels normal. Two years later, after a second pregnancy, the problem recurs.

Understanding the disease

Postpartum and silent thyroiditis are most likely variations of the same disease. Postpartum thyroiditis occurs usually three to six months after a pregnancy, while silent thyroiditis can happen to anyone at any time.

This disease is classed as an autoimmune disorder because high levels of peroxidase autoantibodies are found in the blood (refer to Chapter 4). In this condition, the antibodies seem to damage thyroid cells, causing a release of thyroid hormone that leads to temporary hyperthyroidism. So far, scientists have not managed to link any single gene with this form of thyroiditis.

Postpartum thyroiditis is very common; it occurs after 5–10 per cent of all pregnancies. With this condition, unlike subacute thyroiditis, a new mother has no symptoms of fever or weakness, although she may complain of feeling warm. A rapid heartbeat and palpitations are part of the condition. The thyroid itself is not painful, although it's often abnormally large. The changes that occur in thyroid function are similar to those that occur with subacute thyroiditis, however. First hyperthyroidism occurs, followed by normal function, followed by hypothyroidism. The hypothyroidism may resolve, but the person can develop permanent hypothyroidism.

Women who develop postpartum thyroiditis show a high rate of recurrence in later pregnancies, and 25 per cent of them are permanently hypothyroid after three to five years. As many as 50 per cent of women are hypothyroid seven to nine years after pregnancy. The recurrence rate of silent thyroiditis is also very high.

Ten per cent of women with postpartum thyroiditis experience depression. Therefore, testing thyroid function in any woman complaining of postpartum depression is important.

Interpreting lab results

The lab test that best distinguishes someone with subacute thyroiditis from a person with postpartum or silent thyroiditis is the test of erythrocyte sedimentation rate (ESR). This test measures how quickly the blood cells in a thin column of a person's blood settle down to the bottom – simply a measure of the stickiness of that person's blood due to the presence of inflammatory substances. With subacute thyroiditis, the ESR is high, but with postpartum or silent thyroiditis, the rate is normal.

Thyroid function tests from people with postpartum or silent thyroiditis are initially high, then normal, then low. As in subacute thyroiditis, the hyperthyroid phase of the disease is due to leakage from the thyroid. Because the ratio of T4 to T3 is much higher in the thyroid than in the blood, the ratio of T4 to T3 temporarily becomes high in the blood as well. The TSH and the radioactive uptake of iodine are also on the low side during the hyperthyroid phase.

Getting treatment

Treatment for postpartum and silent thyroiditis depends on the stage at which the disease is diagnosed. If someone is diagnosed during the hyperthyroid phase, she is given the beta-blocker propranolol, which helps to control the symptoms of hyperthyroidism. Antithyroid drugs aren't useful in this case because they won't prevent hyperthyroidism due to the leakage of thyroid hormone. When the hypothyroidism phase occurs, thyroid hormone replacement is given with the understanding that it probably isn't needed on a permanent basis.

Identifying Acute Thyroiditis

Patrick is a 45-year-old man who suddenly develops severe pain in his neck, fever, and chills. The pain is so severe that he has to bend his neck forward to cope with it. He can't swallow without pain. He also feels weak.

Patrick goes off to see his doctor, who notes that he is very sick. His thyroid gland is extremely tender, and he has a fever. The doctor sends him urgently to the thyroid specialist clinic, where the consultant notes that the tender area is somewhat soft. He puts a fine needle into the area and removes a quantity of pus. The pus is sent for culture and for staining to determine which type of bacteria is causing the infection, and Patrick is placed on an antibiotic, along with aspirin.

In a few days, Patrick is feeling much better. The pus grows a type of bacterium that is sensitive to the antibiotic used, and this medication is continued for 10 days. Patrick recovers fully.

Acute thyroiditis is much rarer than subacute thyroiditis but is easily confused with subacute, depending on the way the disease appears in the patient. Most doctors will only see a few cases during their working life.

Describing the disease

Many different organisms can infect the thyroid gland to cause acute thyroiditis. Bacteria are present about 70 per cent of the time. The type of bacteria found varies from pneumococcus (which often causes pneumonia) to streptococcus (associated with strep throat) and staphylococcus (which causes skin infections). About 15 per cent of the time, a fungus is the infecting organism; tuberculosis is the cause 10 per cent of the time, and various other bugs are the culprits much less frequently.

Besides the tender thyroid, nearby structures such as the trachea (air passage), larynx (voice box), and oesophagus (swallowing tube) are inflamed, and local lymph glands in the neck are tender. In many people, a connection from the outside (such as the throat) to the thyroid tissue is found, through which the infection invades. This tiny, abnormal opening is called a *fistula* and is a result of a developmental defect that is present from birth. A fistula results when the thyroid tissue moves from the back of the tongue down into the neck (check out Chapter 3 for more on how the thyroid gland develops in a embryo) and acts as an open pipe to the thyroid through which infections can pass. If a fistula is found in association with acute thyroiditis, the fistula is always removed as infection will inevitably recur. In fact, infection of the thyroid is so rare that a fistula is actively sought in every case.

Someone with acute thyroiditis looks obviously sick. The individual complains of a pain in the neck and may have to bend her neck forward to decrease it. She has a fever and chills. The thyroid is enlarged (usually on one side), hot, and tender. Depending on how large the thyroid gets, the patient may have trouble swallowing or even breathing. Lymph nodes are often enlarged, swollen, and tender as well.

Confirming the diagnosis with lab tests

In a person with acute thyroiditis, general blood tests for infection, such as the white blood cell count and the erythrocyte sedimentation rate, are abnormally high. These results confirm that an infection or inflammation is present.

When thyroid tests such as the free T4 and the TSH are done, the results are generally normal, although once in a while the destruction of the thyroid is so great that enough hormone leaks to cause hyperthyroidism. Thyroid uptake of radioactive iodine is normal, and thyroid autoantibodies are negative.

The best test for acute thyroiditis is a needle biopsy. Usually, the biopsy shows inflammation and the infecting organism, but occasionally, no inflammation is seen. Then the diagnosis is much more difficult. Sometimes the thyroid has an abscess, which is drained via the needle.

Treating acute thyroiditis

The treatment for this condition is to give the appropriate antibiotic based upon the suspected organism. The biopsy can provide a good idea of what type of organism is causing the infection, which is later confirmed from a culture of the biopsy tissue. The right antibiotic generally cures the infection and restores normal thyroid function. Sometimes the infection does not respond, and surgery to remove the infected part of the thyroid or the whole thyroid is necessary.

When acute thyroiditis recurs, this event suggests that a fistula is allowing bacteria to get into the thyroid from the outside. In that situation, the person has a barium swallow test, during which X-rays show a trail of barium going from the throat into the thyroid gland. Surgery is then required to eliminate the fistula.

Occasionally, acute thyroiditis causes such damage to the thyroid tissue that hypothyroidism results, and treatment with replacement thyroid hormone is needed.

Diagnosing a Rare Form of Thyroiditis

Christopher is a 42-year-old man who comes to his doctor complaining of gaining weight and feeling tired, weak, cold, and sleepy. He also says that his neck feels very tight. He has trouble swallowing and breathing.

His doctor examines him and notes that his neck feels very dense. His thyroid barely moves when he swallows. The doctor does not feel swelling in the lymph nodes in his neck.

The doctor runs thyroid function tests, which show a low free T4 and a high TSH. At the same time, he obtains a calcium level, and this test result is low as well. A test of the hormone made in the parathyroid glands called parathyroid hormone is run, and the result of that test is low. The doctor refers Chris to the thyroid specialist clinic where a barium swallow shows compression on the oesophagus. The consultant attempts to do a fine needle biopsy of Chris's thyroid, but is unable to get tissue. The doctor makes a presumptive diagnosis of Riedel's thyroiditis, and starts Chris on treatment with corticosteroids, thyroid hormone, and calcium. Chris's symptoms gradually decrease, but the hypothyroidism and the hypoparathyroidism (low parathyroid function resulting in low calcium) remain. Chris continues to take thyroid hormone replacement and vitamin D for the rest of his life.

This final form of thyroiditis is included for completeness, although it's so rare that most doctors will not come across the condition during their career. The disease is called *Riedel's thyroiditis* and its cause is unknown. The condition is associated with elevated levels of antithyroid autoantibodies so autoimmunity is probably playing some role, especially in view of the good response to corticosteroids. Some specialists believe that Riedel's thyroiditis is a variant of chronic autoimmune thyroiditis (refer to Chapter 5). Both conditions are associated with autoantibodies and both are often associated with other autoimmune diseases in the same person.

Riedel's thyroiditis is probably twice as frequent in men as in women, but as so few cases are recorded it's hard to tell. It tends to occur between ages 30 and 60.

First, the thyroid develops fibrosis – the replacement of thyroid tissue by hard fibres – that is often so dense that thyroid function is lost and the patient becomes hypothyroid. The fibrous tissue firmly attaches the thyroid to the trachea and the nearby muscles so that it doesn't move in the neck. Even a small needle can't penetrate the woody, fibrous tissue, so fine needle aspiration biopsy is impossible.

If the fibrosis continues, it involves the parathyroid glands, which sit behind the thyroid. If these glands are destroyed, the patient also develops hypoparathyroidism. Because the parathyroid glands are important for maintaining calcium levels, the result of this disease is a fall in calcium. Symptoms of tingling and numbness in the hands and feet and tingling around the mouth begin to occur. As the calcium falls, it can result in severe muscle spasms.

Sometimes, the fibrosis stops and the person remains stable. Other times, it continues to cause trouble with breathing, swallowing, and even talking.

When the doctor does thyroid function tests early in the disease, they are often normal. Later, the patient becomes hypothyroid, although the erythrocyte sedimentation rate remains normal.

Because the fibrosis is so invasive, Riedel's thyroiditis is sometimes confused with anaplastic carcinoma, an extremely rapid-growing, invasive form of thyroid cancer (refer to Chapter 8). A biopsy generally shows the difference, but sometimes the condition is not recognised until the patient is in the operating room about to have surgery for what the surgeon thinks is cancer.

If severe neck symptoms occur, surgery is sometimes necessary to free up the tissues. Sometimes, so much fibrosis is present that surgery isn't successful in removing the tissue. A trial of corticosteroids often slows or stops progression of the disease. The other agent that has shown some success is the anti-oestrogen drug, tamoxifen.

Chapter 12

Overcoming Iodine Deficiency Disease

. . . .

. . . .

*I*n the movie *Love and Death,* Woody Allen describes a convention of village idiots in Russia. If such a convention actually occurred, sadly, most of the people in attendance would probably have iodine deficiency disease.

As you discover in this chapter, iodine deficiency disease is the world's most common and preventable cause of impaired mental ability. What stops it from elimination is more often politics than medicine. The situation is very similar to the problem of infectious diseases that are preventable with immunisation. The science of the condition is clearly understood, including the treatment. What's missing is the means to transfer that knowledge into action.

A case in point is the story of the former East Germany. Prior to 1980, 50 per cent of East German adolescents developed *goitres*. A goitre is an enlargement of the thyroid that's sometimes debilitating. In 1980, the country started to add minute amounts of iodine to common table salt, and the percentage of adolescents with goitre dropped to less than 1 per cent. Unfortunately, with the reunification of Germany, iodisation became voluntary, and the goitre rate began to rise again.

This chapter gives you a greater appreciation of the major role of thyroid hormone in the growth and development of the human body, particularly mental development. When you finish this chapter, you won't have any chance of getting invited to that convention in Russia.

Realising the Vastness of the Problem

More than one-quarter of the world's population suffers from some level of iodine deficiency disease. That portion works out at 1.6 billion people. Of these people, 655 million have a goitre, 26 million have brain damage, and 6 million of those 26 million are classed as 'cretins' – a somewhat unfortunate term, which means that the individuals are so handicapped due to their thyroid condition that they're completely dependent upon those around them to live. Some researchers estimate that for each day we delay treating this vast problem, 50,000 more infants are born with decreased mental capacity due entirely to iodine deficiency.

The reason so many people suffer with this condition is that the food they eat contains little or no iodine, mostly because the ground on which it's farmed is depleted of iodine. Chapter 3 explains that iodine is required to form thyroxine (T4) and triiodothyronine (T3), the two major thyroid hormones – in fact, this requirement is the only known function of iodine in the body.

All the earth's soil used to contain iodine. However, hundreds of thousands of years have seen iodine leached out of the soil in two major areas of the earth: The high mountains and the plains that were covered with fresh water in the past, which were far away from oceans. The high mountains were once covered with glaciers. As the glaciers melted, they carried iodine out of the soil, back to the ocean. In the same way, the flooded plains leached iodine from the soil and carried it back to the ocean as the water flowed away. As a result, high mountains and plains far from oceans are the areas where iodine deficiency disease is most often found.

Crops that grow in such soil are iodine deficient, as are the animals that feed on these crops. If the animal is a cow that provides milk, children who drink that milk are at risk of iodine deficiency. The meat from that cow is also iodine deficient. The result is a huge public health problem. Even pets such as dogs become iodine deficient.

If you look at a map of the world that shows the areas where iodine deficiency disease is most prevalent, you see that vast areas of China, Russia, Mexico, South America, and Africa are rife with the disease. Surprisingly, even developed countries such as the United Kingdom are not spared. In fact, Derbyshire Neck was at one time the common name for a goitre, as iodine deficiency was so common in this part of England. The iodisation of salt and cattle feed helped to solve the problem, but with the current health advice to cut back on salt intake, concern is growing that the problem may recur. In the United States, for example, nearly 12 per cent of people in one study showed evidence of low iodine levels, compared with only 3 per cent 20 years earlier. Recent studies among Europeans show decreases in iodine intake as well.

How iodine deficiency is measured

To determine whether iodine deficiency is present in large populations, the development of simple tools to measure a lack of iodine is necessary. One technique is to measure the amount of iodine excreted in urine. In areas where iodine is not deficient, the iodine in the urine is 100 micrograms per day or more.

If a country or population undertakes an iodisation programme, this urine test is carried out on a sample of the population before they receive iodine, and again at intervals afterwards to see whether the programme is working. (If it is, a much higher level of iodine appears in the urine after iodisation begins.)

The second important measure of iodine deficiency is the frequency of goitres. Traditionally, a goitre is diagnosed if the lobes of the thyroid are larger than the end parts of the thumbs of the person concerned. (These parts are called the *terminal phalanges* of the thumbs.) Unfortunately, such a measurement of the thyroid is hard to make in practise, especially for small children in whom it's most important. To overcome this difficulty, doctors use a portable ultrasound device (refer to Chapter 4), which produces a measurement that is highly accurate and reproducible.

Finally, measurement of thyroid hormones and TSH in the blood helps to evaluate the production of thyroid hormones.

Facing the Consequences of Iodine Lack

If your body lacks iodine, it can't produce sufficient thyroid hormone. This deficiency has severe consequences at every stage of life. This section discusses the price paid in poor health and abnormal function at every stage of life, beginning with a pregnant woman and her baby.

Pregnancy

Even before pregnancy, a lack of T4 hormone appears to affect fertility. Women who are hypothyroid have greater difficulties becoming pregnant, and they have more miscarriages and stillbirths than women with normal thyroid function.

A foetus (developing baby) doesn't begin to make thyroid hormone until the 24th week of pregnancy. Until then, it's dependent upon the mother's T4. During this time, the foetal brain is developing, and the entire chain of events that produces a normal brain requires T4 at every stage. If this hormone is lacking, the consequences are severe.

If a foetus is deficient in T4, this need triggers an increase in the amount of the enzyme that converts T4 to T3 within the brain. This form of the enzyme is not found in other tissues, so the brain is partially protected from hypothyroidism while the rest of the body is not.

The entire body's formation is dependent upon adequate T4. If sufficient hormone is not available, congenital anomalies may occur and the infant may not survive much past birth. If it does, the infant may not live more than a few years. In this nuclear age, it's important to realise that a thyroid gland that is not making enough thyroid hormone will take up large amounts of iodine from whatever source it can. In the case of a nuclear accident, where radioactive iodine is released, a hypothyroid mother will concentrate the iodine and pass it on to her growing foetus. If radioactive iodine does not completely destroy the developing foetal thyroid, that thyroid is very prone to develop thyroid cancer in the future.

Infancy

A new baby deprived of iodine has a goitre and shows signs of hypothyroidism. Depending upon the severity of the lack, the baby may have cretinism, which this chapter explains later on. The brain of a newborn continues to develop up to the age of two years, so giving adequate amounts of iodine immediately after birth may help to prevent problems with mental development. A baby lacking in iodine also shows increased susceptibility to radioactive iodine (or any iodine) and is therefore more vulnerable if exposed to increased levels as a result of a nuclear accident such as occurred in Chernobyl.

Childhood

Iodine-deficient children often have goitres. Their intelligence is usually affected, their motor function (muscle control) is poor and they are sometimes deaf. Like infants, these children have a tendency to accumulate iodine from any source and are at greater risk in the case of a nuclear accident.

Adulthood

After an iodine-deficient child grows up, he often has a goitre if they develop into an iodine-deficient adult, though not always. He usually has special intellectual needs, and may have movement difficulties. This person's thyroid gland is highly susceptible to radioactivity.

The costs of iodine deficiency disorder are enormous both for the individual and for society.

Endemic Cretinism

Shabmir is a 46-year-old woman living in Pakistan. She has a huge growth on the front of her neck that the doctors tell her is a goitre. She isn't alone, because more than 70 per cent of the villagers around her suffer from the same condition.

Shabmir has little aptitude for learning and, because of the unsightly growth on her neck, she is discriminated against by those who do not have the same problem (perhaps because they come from an area with sufficient iodine in the food). Not only that, the goitre is so large that she has difficulty moving her head and neck, which makes earning a living difficult. Her husband also has a severe goitre, which is the only reason he agreed to marry her.

Shabmir is unable to have a baby. The one time she finds she is pregnant, the baby is stillborn. She does not manage to get pregnant again.

She appears swollen and lethargic. She has little interest in her neighbours or her surroundings, and she tends to sleep a lot.

Shabmir's story is typical of the way that iodine deficiency disease affects the lives of millions of people. Whole populations are rendered unable to function by this worldwide plague. A village of people with iodine deficiency disease is unable to govern itself or provide an economic base to help better the condition of the people, or to take the steps necessary to overcome the problem, including using iodine. The shame is that this condition is completely preventable.

This section describes the different ways that iodine deficiency disease appears in people. The manifestations of iodine deficiency disease are far worse than the hypothyroidism commonly found in the United Kingdom (refer to Chapter 5) because the hypothyroidism associated with lack of iodine begins when babies are conceived. Their mothers are already hypothyroid. Unless and until the chain of iodine deficiency is broken with the provision of sufficient iodine, the disease continues to disrupt the lives of a quarter of the world's population.

Endemic cretinism is the term used for the group of signs and symptoms that are found when severe iodine deficiency affects a significant proportion of a population. Endemic cretinism consists of several features:

- More than 5 per cent of children age 6 to 12 have enlarged thyroid glands associated with endemic goitre.

- Those affected have problems with mental function and show either

  - Predominantly nervous system symptoms (such as defects of hearing and speech) as well as problems with standing and walking, which is called *nervous cretinism*, or

  - Symptoms of hypothyroidism and reduced growth called *myxoedematous cretinism*

- In areas where iodine is adequately replaced, cretinism does not occur.

Figure 12-1 shows a typical goitre on a person living in an area of endemic cretinism.

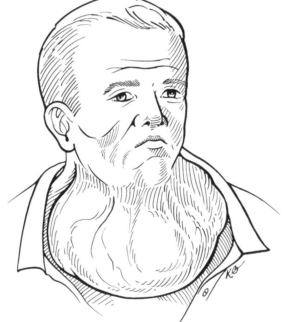

Figure 12-1: A typical goitre on a person living in an area of endemic cretinism.

Looking at the geographic distribution

Endemic cretinism is found in the mountain regions of the world, as explained earlier in this chapter. The condition is most commonly found in the Andes and the Himalayas. It occurred in the Alps until iodine replacement began several decades ago, but areas do still exist there where people don't get sufficient iodine. Endemic cretinism is found in mountainous regions of China, the Pacific, and the Middle East, and in lowlands away from the ocean where heavy rains wash iodine out of the soil. The condition is also present in central Africa, in central Brazil, and even in Holland.

In Europe, iodine deficiency disease remains a significant problem in numerous countries, including: Austria, Belgium, Bulgaria, Russia and some of the former Soviet States, Croatia, Germany, Greece, Holland, Hungary, Ireland, Portugal, Romania, Spain, and Turkey.

Australia has the problem of endemic cretinism in its mountainous regions, especially Tasmania.

In South Asia, iodine deficiency disease is common in Bangladesh, India, Nepal, Tibet, and Pakistan.

In Southeast Asia, large populations of people with goitres are found in Burma, Vietnam, Thailand, and New Guinea.

In Central and South America, large populations lack iodine in Bolivia, Brazil, Chile, Ecuador, Mexico, Peru, and Venezuela – mostly in the Andes Mountains and the mountains of Mexico.

In Africa, endemic cretinism is found in Cameroon, the Central African Republic, Nigeria, Uganda, Rwanda, the Sudan, Tanzania, Zaire, and Zimbabwe.

Contributing factors

Lack of iodine is, without a doubt, the main factor in endemic cretinism, but other issues definitely play a role in different areas of the world. Dietary factors other than iodine consumption are a major aspect of iodine deficiency disease.

In some areas of iodine deficiency disease, the normal diet includes substances that are harmful to the thyroid. In Africa, for example, cassava is a major part of the diet – cassava is a starchy tuberous tree root often used in cooking in the form of flour. Cassava contains cyanide, which is destroyed only if the food is properly prepared. If not, the cyanide is converted into thiocyanate in the body. Thiocyanate competes with iodine for uptake in the thyroid; thus, decreasing even further the tiny amount of iodine that gets into the thyroid. (If someone consumes sufficient iodine, it overcomes any block from thiocyanate.)

Soy beans also interfere with thyroid function, preventing the production of thyroid hormone in the thyroid gland (check out Chapter 10). Again, sufficient iodine can overcome the block and permit normal production of thyroid hormone, but when iodine is scarce, this extra loss of thyroid hormone makes a huge difference.

A third group of foods that contribute to endemic cretinism is the *Brassica* group of vegetables, which includes foods such as broccoli and cauliflower. Hypothyroidism is more common in areas where these vegetables make up a large part of the diet and the diet is deficient in iodine.

Other foods that impair thyroid hormone production and are significant sources of food calories in certain areas of the world are

- Bamboo shoots
- Sweetcorn
- Lima beans
- Sweet potatoes

Another important contributing factor in the development of iodine deficiency disease is the absence of another trace element, selenium, in the diet in certain areas, especially in China, Siberia, Korea, Tibet, and Central Africa. These places are where iodine deficiency is already present. Selenium is a mineral that the body needs in order to create the enzyme that turns T4 into the more potent T3.

In fact, selenium plays an important role in reducing the number of goitres associated with iodine deficiency. The enzyme in the thyroid that selenium helps to produce also has the function of disposing of hydrogen peroxide, a side product of thyroid hormone production. When selenium is lacking, a build up of hydrogen peroxide may destroy thyroid cells, leading to a small thyroid. This small thyroid is still not healthy, however, despite the lack of a goitre.

When both selenium and iodine are absent from the diet, a condition called *Kashin–Beck disease* develops. This disease can lead to short stature as a result of the destruction of the growth-plates at the ends of the long bones. The damage is different than that seen in the short stature associated with myxoedematous cretinism, which this chapter describes later.

Goitre: The body's defence

The thyroid and the rest of the body do what they can to prevent hypothyroidism. The first response is a fall in the production of T4 (refer to Chapter 3 for more on T3 and T4). When this drop occurs, the pituitary gland doesn't sense sufficient T3 in the brain and responds by secreting more TSH (refer to Chapter 3). The thyroid reacts by getting larger – thus, forming a goitre – and by making more of the active hormone T3 (relative to the amount of T4). At the same time, the body converts more T4 into T3 away from the thyroid.

If the intake of iodine is severely limited, T3 production starts to fall. The consequence is severe hypothyroidism, which is particularly damaging to the brain.

Neurologic cretinism

The belief is that neurologic cretinism results from a lack of thyroid hormone from the mother during the period of the third to the sixth month of pregnancy. The severe lack of iodine means that the growing foetus is unable to make thyroid hormone, either. During this time period, the brain needs enough thyroid hormone to develop the ability to hear as well as perform important motor (movement) functions, which are the abilities most affected in this form of cretinism.

Neurologic cretinism has three major characteristics:

- Mental impairment, although memory and social functions are unaffected

- Deafness and often loss of speech

- Stiffness of the arms and legs and an increase in the reflexes (opposite to what is expected in hypothyroidism). The result is that this individual has a shuffling gait or is unable to walk at all.

A person affected by neurologic cretinism may not develop hypothyroidism later in life. If that person receives sufficient iodine, their thyroid makes sufficient thyroid hormone. But, sadly, the damage due to the lack of thyroid hormone during development of the brain is irreversible.

Myxoedematous cretinism

People with myxoedematous cretinism are not as mentally impaired as those with neurologic cretinism. They aren't usually deaf or mute as a result of their condition. Instead, they demonstrate the signs and symptoms of severe hypothyroidism from birth, including:

- Very dry, scaly, and thickened skin
- Reduced growth

✔ Thin hair, eyelashes, and eyebrows

✔ Puffy features

✔ Delayed sexual maturation

People with this condition do not have enlarged thyroids, but their thyroids are often replaced with scar tissue. As a result, their uptake of radioactive iodine is reduced despite having very high TSH levels. The levels of T4 and T3 hormones are very low. Many individuals have a combination of these two conditions.

Just why such a difference exists between the two conditions isn't clear, although a study published in 1988 sheds some light on this subject. In Qinghai Province in China, researchers found people with both neurological and myxoedematous cretinism along with a mixed group that showed signs of both conditions. The difference between the types of cretinism is explainable by the length of time that these individuals were hypothyroid after birth; those people with myxoedematous cretinism appear to suffer hypothyroidism for a longer time than those with neurologic cretinism.

Individuals with neurologic cretinism develop mental impairment from a lack of thyroid hormone during brain development, but then get enough iodine to produce normal amounts of thyroid hormone after they are born. So, individuals with myxoedematous cretinism show signs of thyroid destruction, while those people with neurologic cretinism have normal thyroid function. The conclusion of the researchers is that these two disorders are actually the same, only modified according to the amount of hypothyroidism experienced after birth.

Managing the Problem of Iodine Deficiency

You may think that managing the problem of iodine deficiency disease – preventing all goitres, cretinism, thyroid-related physical and mental impairment, plus hypothyroidism – is relatively easy. The trick is just to get everyone to eat sufficient iodine. The adult daily requirement is just 150 micrograms of iodine – which amounts to a mere, microscopic pinch. Over the lifetime of an individual, only a teaspoon of iodine is required. But consuming enough iodine is much easier said than done. And sufficient iodine consumption must occur prior to the conception of a baby in order to prevent the occurrence of cretinism.

A sprinkle of salt

The richest food source of iodine is seafood (fish, crustaceans, seaweed) and, to a lesser extent, milk, eggs, and meat. Fruits and vegetables contain very little iodine. Using iodine-rich foods to solve the problem is not possible, though, as diets and tastes differ throughout the world, and the logistics of transporting sufficient daily amounts of fish, milk, eggs, or meat to everyone in the world are overwhelming.

Iodisation in Bangladesh

The history of efforts to overcome iodine deficiency disease in Bangladesh serves as an excellent illustration of the problems that are encountered. Research shows that only 55 per cent of households in Bangladesh consume iodised salt, despite international efforts to rid the nation of iodine deficiency.

Bangladesh is subject to annual flooding with monsoon rains that effectively wash all iodine out of the soil. The iodine washes into the Bay of Bengal, which means that fish caught there contain plenty of iodine. However, most of the population of the country lives in rural areas far away from the supply of iodine. As a result, more than 50 million people in Bangladesh have goitres.

Since 1984, a Law of Iodination makes the selling of salt in Bangladesh without it being iodised illegal, although penalties for this only came into force in 1992. The cost of iodised salt in Bangladesh is 14 pence per kilogram, while non-iodised salt is 8 pence per kilogram, so the poorest families buy the cheaper salt.

The cost of iodising salt is less than 3 pence per person per year. The process is very simple, carried out in a salt factory. But tests of iodine in salt show that as many as half the factories in Bangladesh are producing salt with insufficient iodine. In a country with a population the size of Bangladesh, this amount represents inadequate iodine intake for millions of people.

Some of the so-called iodised salt is not iodised at all in Bangladesh so that the provider can make an extra profit. Salt is sometimes brought in from other countries, mislabelled as iodised, and sold for a cheaper price than Bangladesh iodised salt. Bangladesh borders on Myanmar (formerly Burma) and India, countries that are not as strict in enforcing iodisation. So smuggling contributes to iodine deficiency disease in Bangladesh as well.

One step in the right direction is the development of a simple kit by UNICEF (The United Nations Children's Fund) that detects whether salt contains iodine. A drop of liquid solution added to salt turns the salt blue if iodine is present. These kits are distributed to school children, who test their salt at home.

You can see that a successful iodisation programme involves much more than passing a law and setting up salt iodisation processing in salt factories. A mountain of barriers can block such a simple solution.

Because virtually every culture in the world uses salt, which is cheap and simple to iodise, iodised salt is the standard way of overcoming the problem of iodine deficiency disease. The amount of salt needed to carry the daily requirement of 150 micrograms of iodine is very small and easily consumed.

In many countries, salt iodisation works well, but in some areas the goal of eliminating iodine deficiency disease is not yet achieved.

One major organisation, the International Council for the Control of Iodine Deficiency Disorders (ICCIDD), serves as the central organisation for coordination efforts worldwide. This organisation has a global iodised salt logo, which manufacturers place on packages of salt that are properly iodised (see Figure 12-2).

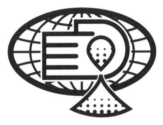

Figure 12-2:
The global iodised salt logo.

An injection of oil

A highly effective way of managing iodine deficiency disorder is to inject iodised oil into the muscle of iodine deficient people. This substance is called Lipiodol, and a single injection provides enough iodine to last for four years or longer. An oral form of Lipiodol is also available, but it lasts little more than a year when taken this way. Iodine given through this oil can significantly shrink goitres in just a few months. However, giving iodine injections also has its problems.

Iodine deficiency is found in rural areas where administering sterile injections is not always possible. Similarly, qualified people are not always available to give the injections. Sufficient supplies of sterile needles and the iodised oil are needed and, in this age of acquired immune deficiency syndrome (AIDS), many people are reluctant to accept an injection. The oral form of Lipiodol, of course, solves all these problems.

A slice of bread or cup of water

Other ways of managing iodine deficiency that are effective in some areas include the iodisation of bread and the addition of iodine to the water supply. The problem with the iodisation of bread is that bread consumption varies widely, and so this method works only in limited areas. Adding iodine to water doesn't work in areas with no public water supply, as is the case in most areas of the world where iodine deficiency disease is most prevalent.

Drawbacks of Iodisation

One major problem that occurs when iodisation programmes are undertaken is the occurrence of hyperthyroidism when a lot of iodine is given to a person whose thyroid is under hyperstimulation with TSH. This happens with iodine injections and even with iodised salt that contains excessive iodine. The tools for managing hyperthyroidism (refer to Chapter 6) in a rural environment are not always readily available, especially when dealing with a large number of cases.

Chapter 13

Going In: Surgery on the Thyroid Gland

. . . .

In This Chapter

▶ Deciding whether you need surgery

▶ Picking the surgeon

▶ Preparing for surgery

▶ Understanding the procedure

▶ Managing after surgery

. . . .

*I*f you need a thyroid operation, the good news is that the thyroid is in a very convenient location. Positioned just a few millimetres beneath the skin of your neck, your thyroid gland is easily found. Except in rare circumstances in which the gland is matted down with fibrosis (check out Chapter 11 for more on *Riedel's thyroiditis*) and difficult to free up, thyroid surgery is relatively simple in the hands of a skilled surgeon. Complications are few and infrequent, and the result of surgery is usually very satisfactory.

If you are about to have surgery, you need to know a few things to make the experience as benign as possible. Revealing those things is the purpose of this chapter. Although you won't be an expert on thyroid surgery after reading this information (at least not after your first reading), you will get a good idea of what to expect, so that you won't get any surprises.

Deciding When Surgery Is Necessary

John is a 45-year-old man who has a solitary thyroid nodule – a lump on the thyroid. His GP checks his thyroid function tests, which come back normal, and immediately refers John to the thyroid specialist clinic. The consultant endocrinologist (hormone expert) performs a fine needle biopsy, which shows a follicular lesion – tissue that looks like normal thyroid follicles (the circles of cells that make thyroid hormone). The pathologist is uncertain whether the nodule is cancerous or not. The consultant arranges for John to see a thyroid surgeon with extensive experience, to discuss thyroid surgery. After examining John, the surgeon tells him that he needs a lobectomy (the removal of one lobe of the thyroid). During the operation, a pathologist will examine the tissue that is removed to give a definitive diagnosis. If the lobectomy shows that John has follicular cancer, the surgeon plans to remove the whole thyroid gland (total thyroidectomy). If the tissue is benign, the surgeon plans to leave the remaining lobe intact.

John doesn't eat on the morning of surgery. The operation is supposed to start at 9a.m., but due to various glitches, it doesn't begin until 11a.m. He is given a general anaesthetic and the operation goes smoothly. The pathologist examines the excised thyroid tissue under a microscope and diagnoses a follicular carcinoma (cancer) so the surgeon proceeds to a total thyroidectomy. The surgeon cannot feel enlarged lymph nodes on the side of the thyroid, but removes nodes in the central neck to look for cancer there. The pathologist determines that these nodes are not cancerous.

After the surgery, John feels some soreness in his neck but is not hoarse. The incision on his neck is covered with a clear plastic bandage. John has a chest X-ray and bone scan to make certain that cancer hasn't spread to those areas. These tests come back negative, indicating no cancer spread.

Several weeks after surgery, John receives a dose of radioactive iodine (refer to Chapter 6) to destroy any remaining thyroid tissue. For the next several years, John sees his doctor about every six months. The doctor finds no indications that the cancer is recurring.

A number of reasons might bring you to the thyroid surgeon. John's situation is one of the most serious – thyroid cancer (check out Chapter 8 for more on the types and treatment of thyroid cancer). But several other thyroid situations are best handled with surgery as well.

If you are hyperthyroid and antithyroid pills don't successfully treat your condition (or if you're allergic to them), and you don't want to have treatment with radioactive iodine, surgery is your only other choice. If you're pregnant and develop hyperthyroidism, and you're unable to take the antithyroid pills because of allergies, surgery is your only option. (You cannot receive radioactive iodine during pregnancy as this treatment harms your baby's thyroid tissue, too.)

If you have a large thyroid that's causing local symptoms in your neck, such as trouble swallowing or breathing, or if the goitre is especially unattractive, surgery is necessary, although radioactive iodine is another option in these situations.

Talking Things Over

National guidelines from the British Thyroid Association and the Royal College of Physicians of London recommend that, if you have symptoms that might be due to thyroid cancer, your doctor refers you to a thyroid specialist clinic. This clinic is run by a team that includes an experienced thyroid surgeon, as well as a thyroid or endocrine physician, pathologist, oncologist (cancer specialist) and a nuclear medicine expert, as well as highly trained nurses. The clinic aims to see you as soon as possible and, if you have a thyroid lump, you're usually seen within two weeks of referral.

When you need surgery, the thyroid specialist clinic understands that you have a lot of important questions that need to be fully discussed before going ahead with surgery. Trained nurses are available in the clinic for you to talk to, and you're also given written information about your condition and its treatment. This information is especially important if you are diagnosed with thyroid cancer. In this case, the guidelines also allow you the opportunity for another appointment for further explanations and discussion, as you may find difficulty taking in all the information you're given at a single consultation. When your diagnosis is cancer, the clinic also aims to inform your GP within 24 hours (by telephone or fax) so that she is aware of the situation, and your planned treatment.

If at any time you have questions about your thyroid condition, the operation you need, or your treatment (whether current or future) always ask.

Preparing for Surgery

If you're having an operation for hyperthyroidism, you'll probably take anti-thyroid pills for four to six weeks before surgery to get your thyroid function as normal as possible according to a free T4 test. (If you can't take anti-thyroid pills because of an allergy, obviously you skip this step.) You may also need iodine for 10 days before surgery to reduce the size of the thyroid and the blood vessels supplying it. If you have symptoms such as a rapid heartbeat or shakiness, you can control them with propranolol; a type of drug called a beta-blocker that damps down overactivity in part of your nervous system.

If you have hypothyroidism, you need to take thyroid hormone replacement pills before surgery so that your thyroid function is normal. Anaesthesia is risky if the patient is very hypothyroid.

If you're taking aspirin or other medications like warfarin to thin your blood (and therefore prolong bleeding), you also need to stop taking these a week before surgery. Ask your doctor or surgeon for advice about what to do if they haven't already mentioned this important fact. A few days prior to surgery, you also have blood tests to confirm that your liver and kidneys are performing satisfactorily. The doctor also wants to check that you do not have anaemia (deficiency of red cells or of haemoglobin in your blood), although you won't lose much blood during thyroid surgery.

You should eat nothing after supper the night before surgery. The anxiety, the trauma of surgery, and the anaesthesia all make you more prone to vomit, and you don't want to have anything in your stomach should this happen.

You generally come to the hospital on the morning of surgery. You are wheeled into the operating room, where the anaesthetist gives you a general anaesthetic. (Sometimes you are given a local anaesthetic instead, but this action is unusual.) Two hours later, you wake up minus some of or all your thyroid. (Be aware though that it's not an efficient way to lose weight – unless you have a particularly large goitre.)

What Happens During Surgery

After all the preparations of cleaning and covering the area of the operation, the surgeon makes an incision about 7 to 8 centimetres long horizontally over your thyroid gland. The surgeon carefully places the incision over a normal skin crease (where your skin folds as you bend your head forward) and makes the smallest incision possible to minimise the scar. If the surgeon has to remove lymph nodes, the incision is carried up in the direction of the ear at one or both ends of the incision. The incision cuts through the fat underneath the skin and a thin layer of muscle called the platysma. The skin and the muscle overlying the thyroid are pulled back to reveal the thyroid gland.

The surgeon then sees what he or she needs to deal with in the next hour or so. The thyroid is shaped like a butterfly, with an isthmus (narrow strip) of thyroid tissue connecting the two 'wings' of the butterfly. Above the isthmus, the surgeon may see a projection of thyroid tissue called the pyramidal lobe. This lobe is usually removed during any partial thyroid operation so that it doesn't regrow as a large bump on the front of the neck when the remaining gland enlarges to restore thyroid hormone production.

The surgeon knows that the thyroid is firmly fixed to the trachea (air passage) and larynx (voice box) at the back, so any operation involves freeing up the thyroid before the surgeon removes the thyroid tissue. The surgeon sees two superior thyroid arteries entering the thyroid from above and two inferior thyroid arteries entering the thyroid from below. A fifth artery sometimes enters the thyroid in its central portion from below. These arteries are some-times tied and cut depending upon how much of the thyroid is removed.

The surgeon must also deal with the thyroid veins. The middle thyroid veins connect to the thyroid from the side. These veins are tied and cut. The veins connecting to the top of the thyroid, called the superior thyroid veins, are also tied and cut if the plan is to remove the entire lobe.

Between three and six parathyroid glands, as well as the recurrent laryngeal nerves (one on each side), are found on the back of the thyroid and are care-fully preserved if possible. (See 'Surgical obstacles', the next section, for details.)

Studies show that if a dye is injected into the thyroid, the dye goes to the chain of lymph nodes on the trachea behind the isthmus. The surgeon knows that this chain is where to look first for the spread of cancer.

At this point, the purpose of the surgery determines what's done next. If the operation is to remove a hot nodule (refer to Chapter 7), the surgeon locates any blood supply to it, cuts and ties off the blood supply, and removes the nodule. If hyperthyroidism is the reason for surgery, the surgeon performs a subtotal thyroidectomy, leaving a few grams of the part of the thyroid near-est the trachea to avoid damaging the parathyroid glands. If surgery is for thyroid cancer, the procedure is dependent on the type and spread of the disease. (For more information, refer to Chapter 8 and also see the section 'Extent of surgery' later on in this chapter.)

Surgical obstacles

In any thyroid surgery, the main obstacles to easy surgery are the parathy-roid glands and the recurrent laryngeal nerves.

Parathyroid glands

The parathyroid glands sit on the back of the thyroid and share blood supply with it. Usually, you have four of these tiny glands, but sometimes you have more or less, and to make things interesting for the surgeon, they are found in many locations.

The parathyroids are responsible for managing the calcium level in your blood. If they aren't functioning, your calcium level falls. Someone whose parathyroids are not functioning may experience tingling in her lips and numbness in her hands or feet, or even severe muscle spasms. Sometimes, the trauma of surgery causes the parathyroids to shut off temporarily, but they recover in a few days.

With a total thyroidectomy, preserving the parathyroid glands is often not possible. In that case, they are cut into small pieces and injected back into a muscle, for example in the shoulder, where they seem to function just fine.

If a person has symptoms of low calcium after surgery, the problem is usually managed with oral calcium supplements. Rarely, intravenous calcium is needed. If, through chance, the parathyroids fail to recover their function after surgery, the patient takes vitamin D and calcium for the rest of their life. This is a rare occurrence associated with only 1 in 300 surgeries of the thyroid.

Recurrent laryngeal nerves

The recurrent laryngeal nerves on both sides of the thyroid are major obstacles to the surgeon. Each nerve controls the vocal cord on its side. Both nerves lie close to the thyroid and are easily cut accidentally or included in a knot that is tying off a blood vessel. If the diagnosis is thyroid cancer, one or both of the recurrent laryngeal nerves may already be cancerous, and are therefore sacrificed at the time of surgery.

Sometimes, the recurrent laryngeal nerves are temporarily damaged or bruised during surgery. If so, the person has a hoarse voice for a few days after the operation. If both nerves are damaged, the situation is more serious, and a tracheostomy is often needed so that the patient can breathe. The damage and the hoarseness can remain as a permanent side effect of the surgery.

Damage to a recurrent laryngeal nerve is normally rare. In good hands, damage doesn't occur more often than once for every 250 operations on the thyroid, as the surgeon is careful to look for, and preserve these important structures.

The superior laryngeal nerve is sometimes injured during surgery as well. Damage to this nerve produces milder symptoms than those of recurrent laryngeal loss. Loss of this nerve produces voice fatigue and a decrease in the range of the voice.

Extent of surgery

A debate rages over how much of the gland to remove when a cancer is present in the thyroid. Most of the debate concerns small thyroid cancers – those that measure less than 1.5 centimetres in diameter. The survival rate for this size cancer seems to be just as good whether a total thyroidectomy or less than a total thyroidectomy is done. Less than a total thyroidectomy leaves a small amount of thyroid tissue behind, to protect the recurrent laryngeal nerve on one side.

A total thyroidectomy is an attempt to remove all visible thyroid tissue. The surgery is extensive, more difficult to perform than partial removal of the thyroid, and results in more frequent damage to parathyroids and nerves. Therefore, many surgeons do a near-total thyroidectomy, leaving a small piece of one lobe of the thyroid intact, when the tumour is this small.

Other surgeons elect to do a total thyroidectomy on all thyroid cancer patients. They offer fairly convincing arguments:

- The morbidity and mortality rate of this surgery in their hands is very low.

- Thyroid cancer is often bilateral, meaning that it affects both lobes of the thyroid. If radiation is the cause of cancer, it's almost always bilateral.

- Scanning for evidence of new tumours, and treating any new tumours, is much easier when no thyroid gland remains to take up radioactive iodine.

- After surgery, levels of thyroglobulin in the blood fall to zero. Therefore, if blood tests later show that a patient's thyroglobulin levels are rising, that's a strong indicator that a tumour is recurring.

After all or part of the thyroid is removed, the question arises as to whether to remove lymph nodes, especially if none are enlarged. The British Thyroid Association and the Royal College of Physicians of London guidelines recommend that all lymph nodes in the central compartment of the neck be removed because cancer often spreads there first. Other nodes along the sides of the neck are felt and, if any suspicious nodes are discovered, biopsies are taken and sent for immediate analysis. If the pathologist confirms that the cancer has spread to these nodes, then lymph nodes on the side of the neck are carefully dissected out, too. This procedure is called a *modified radical neck dissection*. A more extensive form of this surgery, called an *unmodified radical neck dissection*, involves removing muscles and other tissues, too. No study has ever shown that this extensive surgery improves mortality rates and, as it leaves the patient disfigured for no reason, is now rarely required.

If surgery is deemed necessary, the surgeon attempts to remove as much cancer and thyroid as possible if the tumour is the undifferentiated (anaplastic) type (refer to Chapter 8). By the time surgery is performed, these tumours usually have already spread, but surgery can sometimes slow the inevitable local spread of this aggressive type of cancer.

A tumour of the medullary type (refer to Chapter 8) is managed with a total thyroidectomy and the removal of the central nodes around the trachea; lateral nodes to the side of the thyroid are removed only if they are visibly enlarged. Medullary tumours often secrete hormones that cause diarrhoea or stimulate the adrenal gland, so removing as much tissue as possible prevents or reverses these complications.

Papillary cancer (refer to Chapter 8) with tumours greater than 1 cm in diameter, plus nodes or secondaries, and those with familial disease or disease due to radioactive exposure, undergo surgery for a total thyroidectomy and local lymph nodes. With a small papillary thyroid cancer of less than 1 centimetre in diameter with no nodes or signs of secondary malignant growths, surgery involves removal of just the thyroid lobe in which the cancer is situated, plus the middle bit of the thyroid (isthmus). This operation is called a *lobectomy* and leaves part of the thyroid intact as the chance that cancer has spread into the other lobe is small.

For follicular cancer (refer to Chapter 8), a lobectomy is performed where the tumour is confined to the thyroid gland.

If a surgeon has any concern about bleeding after surgery, or if so much tissue is removed that a large space is left in the neck, the surgeon leaves a drain in the wound. A drain is needed only rarely and is usually removed after a day or two in any case. The drain helps prevent fluid accumulation and results in a better cosmetic outcome.

Considering a New Approach

Recently, some surgeons are trying a less invasive approach to thyroid surgery called *endoscopic thyroid surgery*. This type of surgery is done when a diagnosis of cancer is uncertain and they just want to remove a nodule for examination under a microscope. A tiny tube is inserted in the neck, and a stream of carbon dioxide gas opens up the area. The surgeon uses high magnification to see the area in excellent anatomical detail. Another tube inserted into the area has a cutting edge that allows for removal of the nodule. The result is a less unsightly scar and a quicker return to activity for most people, although the amount of pain that these patients feel is about the same as for those who have a conventional operation.

This surgery may take a little longer than an open operation. If cancer is found during the endoscopic surgery, the surgeon usually opens the neck to proceed with an open, total thyroidectomy. However, this operation is promising as a way to avoid large scars and shorten the time between surgery and returning to work. As surgeons gain more experience with this method, it may start to replace the open operation.

Possible Complications

The section 'Recurrent laryngeal nerves' earlier in the chapter tells you what happens if you suffer recurrent laryngeal nerve damage or the loss of parathyroid gland function. You need to know about a few other possible complications from thyroid surgery that, although rare, do occur.

One complication is bleeding. If bleeding occurs, it happens in the first few hours after surgery and occasionally prompts the surgeon to go back in and tie off the bleeding vessels. Placing a bandage over the site of the operation is often necessary. If the bandage is too tight and bleeding occurs, the bleeding can compress the trachea and cause breathing difficulties.

Any surgery also opens up the possibility of wound infection, which responds to antibiotics.

Major operations also thicken the blood as a result of inflammation, immobility, and sometimes dehydration. As thickening can lead to unwanted and potentially dangerous blood clots in the deep veins of the legs, steps are taken during the operation to help prevent these deep vein thromboses. The precautions include wearing graduated compression hose (stockings) and the use of pneumatic devices that compress your calves during surgery to stop blood pooling in your legs. In some cases, injections of heparin, which thins the blood, are given as well.

Recuperating After the Operation

Anyone who has had extensive removal of their thyroid needs to take thyroid hormone replacement tablets for the rest of their life. If the operation is for thyroid cancer, you are given enough thyroid hormone to mildly suppress your thyroid-stimulating hormone (TSH).

Most people leave the hospital the same day of the surgery if no complications develop, which is usually the case.

The usual recovery time from the surgery is about a week. During that time, you feel some neck stiffness and tenderness. Your throat is sore and your voice is hoarse. You have a cough for a few days and feel some pain when you swallow. The scar becomes hard initially and then softens over the next few months. Occasionally, a person forms a very thick scar called a *keloid.* Unfortunately, attempts to remove a keloid with plastic surgery often result in new keloid formation. Fortunately, the appearance of most healed scars is improved by applying an adhesive, silicone gel sheet (for example, Cica-Care and Boots Scar Reduction Patches) that flatten, soften, and fade red and raised scars. Another approach is to massage in Rosa Mosqueta oil, which is pressed from the seeds of an Andean wild rose. The oil is exceptionally rich in linoleic and linolenic essential fatty acids that also help to improve the appearance of scars.

The only recommended post-operative restriction is that you should not submerge the wound in water for the first day or two. You can drive a car as soon as your head can turn without difficulty. Many people are back at work in two weeks. The surgeon often wants to see you again about three weeks after surgery to check on your results.

Chapter 14

Exciting New Approaches in Thyroid Treatment

· ·

· ·

*T*his chapter tells you about a selection of the most important discoveries in thyroid medicine during the last few years. Single studies of a subject are sometimes revised or even overturned when someone else does a similar study, so keep an open mind when new (and not necessarily validated) material such as this is presented.

Appendix B in this book points you towards Web site resources that are updated more frequently than is possible for a book, so don't hesitate to make use of these as well.

Preventing Ill Effects of Large Doses of Iodine

Many of the agents that allow radiologists to view the insides of things, such as the bowels, contain a lot of iodine. Just how much does all this iodine affect thyroid function? That uncertainty was what a group from Germany studied and published in the periodical *Endoscopy* in March 2001. They looked at 70 people who didn't have known thyroid disease (TSH normal), all of whom needed a test called – take a deep breath – an *endoscopic retrograde cholangiopancreatogram* or ERCP for short. This study involves placing a tube into the bile duct system and injecting an iodine-containing agent to look for bile stones or other obstructions. Each person gets a large dose of iodine in the process. The thyroid glands of these people were studied with an ultrasound examination (refer to Chapter 4) prior to their bile duct tests, which divided them into four groups based on thyroid gland size and the presence or absence of previously undiagnosed nodules.

The researchers found that the iodine causes a lasting decrease in thyroid-stimulating hormone (TSH), especially in those who have large thyroids with nodules. The free T3 hormone level increased in all of them, but the free T4 level increased particularly in the people with enlarged nodular thyroid glands. The amount of iodine excreted in their urine greatly increased after the test.

The conclusion of the study is that, before giving someone an iodine-containing contrast agent, it is a good idea to evaluate them first with a thyroid ultrasound, rather than relying on TSH measurement. This two-step procedure identifies those at high risk for developing hyperthyroidism as a result of the iodine exposure.

If you need a test that requires you to receive a large dose of iodine, ask your doctor to check your thyroid carefully prior to the test. A thyroid ultrasound is probably the best test to rule out thyroid disease in this situation. The ultrasound can help you and your doctor prepare for the consequences of giving a lot of iodine if you have an abnormal thyroid gland.

Finding Out More about Hypothyroidism

Many recent studies focus on the proper treatment of hypothyroidism. The following sections offer just a sampling of the research carried out in the last few years. (Check out Chapter 5 for the symptoms of hypothyroidism – underactive thyroid function – and what causes it.)

Treating (or not treating) subclinical hypothyroidism

One of the great debates in thyroid management is what to do about subclinical hypothyroidism. This condition is where someone's TSH level is slightly elevated, their free T4 level is normal, and they have some non-specific symptoms that may result from hypothyroidism or something else. Doctors have looked for signs of low thyroid function or a response to thyroid medication in these people, as they are unsure whether or not treatment is necessary.

One study from Italy, published in the *Journal of Clinical Endocrinology and Metabolism* in March 2001, looked at the function of the heart in 20 people with subclinical hypothyroidism, all of whom showed some abnormality in heart activity. Half the study participants were given thyroid treatment, and the other half was given a placebo. The study found that people given the thyroid treatment drug showed an improvement in heart function, while those given a placebo showed no change. The conclusion was that people with subclinical hypothyroidism have measurable abnormalities that are improved with thyroid treatment.

Another study from Germany, published in *Thyroid* in August 2000, looked at heart disease and heart attacks in people with subclinical hypothyroidism. The author found a definite increase in heart disease and heart attacks compared with people without the condition. Various tests of normal heart function, such as changes in heart rate with exercise, indicated that those functions were impaired in people with subclinical hypothyroidism. The most at-risk people were women over the age of 50 who smoked and had elevated TSH levels. Giving thyroid medication improved these functions and also improved the levels of fats in the blood. The author of this study felt that these changes justified the use of thyroid treatment in subclinical hypothyroidism. The author notes, however, that giving a patient replacement thyroid hormone tends to speed up the heart rate and may worsen chest pain, which is an important consideration when treating someone with this condition.

However, researchers at the University of Pennsylvania School of Medicine recently published a paper, in the March 1, 2006 issue of the *Journal of the American Medical Association*, claiming that leaving a mildly underactive thyroid gland untreated does not lead to an increased risk of cardiovascular disease – at least in older people. These scientists measured thyroid function in 3,200 men and women, aged 65 or over, none of whom were taking thyroid hormone replacement. Participants were divided into groups based on their thyroid function and then followed for 13 years. They found that 15 per cent of the study population had a mildly underactive thyroid gland, and that they showed no greater risk of developing a heart attack, stroke, or death from any other cause, than those with normal thyroid function. Of those who had mildly overactive thyroid glands (subclinical hyperthyroidism), 1.5 per cent had an increased risk of developing an abnormal heart rhythm or atrial fibrillation, but even so, they did not have an increased risk of cardiovascular threats such as heart attacks or stroke, either.

Finding the right dose of hormone

A question that keeps coming up among doctors who treat hypothyroidism is 'What is the correct dose of thyroid medication?' Depending on the particular laboratory doing the test, the normal range for TSH is usually 0.3 to 4.5 µU/ml (microunits per millilitre). Some physicians believe that lowering a patient's level of thyroid-stimulating hormone (TSH) to under 5 is sufficient to eliminate signs and symptoms of low thyroid function, but many people still have symptoms at that level. In a study published in the *Medical Journal of Australia* in February 2001, the authors show that lowering the TSH to between 0.3 and 2.0 µU/ml is beneficial.

Against this research, however, is a paper published in the journal *Neurology,* in 2004. Scientists measured the level of TSH in 178 people with Alzheimer's disease and compared their results with 291 people with normal thyroid function. They found that people with Alzheimer's disease have significantly lower levels of TSH and conclude that having a lowered TSH within the normal range is a risk factor of Alzheimer's disease, even when a number of other factors such as smoking are taken into account.

Determining the prevalence of hypothyroidism

How common is thyroid disease in the population? A group in Norway studied this question and published their answer in the *European Journal of Endocrinology,* in November 2000. The group looked at the TSH levels of people who supposedly had no thyroid disease and found that their levels were between 0.49 and 5.7 µU/ml (microunits per millilitre) for females and 0.56 and 4.6 µU/ml for males. By then excluding the people who tested positive for thyroid autoantibodies, which indicates that they are prone to thyroid disease, the range of 'normal' TSH numbers dropped to between 0.49 and 1.9 µU/ml in women. The study did not report the range for the men. The conclusion these researchers arrive at is that despite a huge number of recognised cases of thyroid disease in the population, a significant number of cases are not recognised.

This study offers further proof that the correct normal range for TSH (a range that excludes any person with thyroid disease) is lower than the one quoted by most laboratories.

Linking heart disease and hypothyroidism

A study in *Thyroid* in 1999, pointed out that homocysteine, a substance found in the blood, is an independent risk factor (like high blood pressure, smoking, and high cholesterol) for hardening and furring up of the arteries (atherosclerosis). Because heart disease is commonly found in people with hypothyroidism, the authors of the study measured homocysteine levels in people with clinical hypothyroidism. They found that homocysteine levels were abnormally high, and that these levels fell when the hypothyroidism was treated with thyroid hormone replacement. The authors suggest that the combination of abnormal fats (especially cholesterol) and high levels of homocysteine is the reason that people with clinical hypothyroidism have an increased risk for heart attacks.

A study published in *Endocrine Research* in 2004, found that people with subclinical hypothyroidism have homocysteine levels within the normal range, although when compared with a healthy control group, the difference between them is significant. This discovery suggests that as hypothyroidism worsens, so does the ability to process homocysteine properly.

Recent evidence shows that homocysteine levels are lowered when taking a combination of B-group vitamins, which are involved in processing homocysteine in the body.

A study published in the *Journal of Internal Medicine* in 2003, investigated the relationship between homocysteine levels, B-vitamins, and smoking in 112 people with Graves' disease, both before and after antithyroid therapy. The study found that, in people with hyperthyroidism, homocysteine levels were low, and levels of folate, vitamin B12, and B2 were high. Following antithyroid treatment, homocysteine levels increased while the concentration of B-vitamins decreased significantly. And, for those who smoked, levels of folate and B2 fell significantly lower than for non-smokers. This study also confirms that homocysteine levels increase as levels of B-vitamins decrease. The authors conclude that homocysteine levels change according to thyroid function and are partly attributable to altered blood levels of B-vitamins, particularly in smokers.

If you have hypothyroidism, ask your doctor to measure your homocysteine levels, although this test is not yet routinely available in hospitals. Private laboratories offer the service and you can buy kits to send off a blood sample to measure your homocysteine levels from many pharmacies. Taking a supplement providing folic acid (the synthetic form of folate), B12, B6, and B2 is also a good idea.

Dealing with Hyperthyroidism

Despite the availability of several treatments for hyperthyroidism (see Chapter 6), specialists are not satisfied with any of them. Each treatment is associated with either frequent failure or undesirable side effects like hypothyroidism. The search for better therapy continues.

Measuring calcium levels

A study published in January 2001, emphasises the importance of measuring calcium levels in people with thyroid conditions, especially hyperthyroidism. This German study shows that after thyroid surgery, hypoparathyroidism – the loss of parathyroid function (refer to Chapter 13) – frequently occurs and leads to low calcium levels. In this study, excess parathyroid function was also relatively common in association with thyroid disease, leading to a high calcium level.

Both decreased and increased parathyroid function is found at a higher rate in patients with hyperthyroidism than in people who don't have thyroid disease. If you have hyperthyroidism, ask your doctor to check your calcium levels.

Controlling weight gain

Many people with hyperthyroidism are concerned about getting treatment as they fear they'll gain weight when their thyroid function decreases.

In a study from Edinburgh, Scotland, published in the journal *Thyroid* in December 2000, the authors compare the weight at diagnosis of hyperthyroidism with their weight after normal thyroid function was restored in 43 people given antithyroid drugs, 56 people undergoing thyroid surgery, and 131 people with Graves' disease. The study shows that people who start taking T4 thyroid hormone replacement immediately after their treatment (because they quickly became hypothyroid) gain much less weight than those who did not start taking hormone replacement because their TSH levels were normal.

Harry, the hyperthyroid horse

Hyperthyroidism is managed in a variety of ways. However, for a horse named Harry, surgery was the only consideration. Harry's case was reported in the *Journal of the American Veterinary Medical Association* in October 2000. He suffered from all the symptoms that people show (refer to Chapter 6), including fever, nervousness, and weight loss. His thyroid was prominent, especially on the right side. Harry was treated with surgery to remove the overactive lobe and responded very well.

The authors conclude that defining hypothyroidism using the usual range of TSH after treatment of hyperthyroidism leads to many people not getting the treatment they need. Well-known studies indicate that TSH levels tend to lag behind (remain low) as a person resumes normal thyroid function or even becomes hypothyroid after treatment of hyperthyroidism. In this situation, clinical symptoms and a reduced free T4 level are better indicators of the need for treatment than the TSH level.

Revolutionising thyroid surgery

A new type of thyroid surgery using tiny scopes instead of a large open incision in the neck is suitable for removing thyroid nodules, thyroid lobes and, in some cases, for removing the whole thyroid gland. Some procedures use the gas, carbon dioxide, to raise the skin and gain access to the thyroid gland, via a small incision, while others use a video-assisted, gasless technique. At present, these techniques are suitable for people with small thyroid nodules (less than 35mm) or a small thyroid gland (less than 30ml volume), who have not undergone previous neck surgery. If cancer is found in a nodule, the operation is usually converted into a traditional open-neck surgery for more extensive dissection of lymph nodes. Endoscopic thyroid surgery is rapidly developing and is likely to prove suitable for a wider range of thyroid problems in the near future.

Gathering clues to hyperthyroid eye disease

Just exactly why hyperthyroid eye disease occurs is not clear, but researchers generally believe that the cause is an autoimmune disorder (refer to Chapter 4 for a discussion of thyroid autoantibodies). One suggestion is that thyroglobulin enters the muscles of the eyes, and antibodies react against it. A study from Italy in the journal *Thyroid* in 2001, shows that thyroglobulin is, indeed, found in the muscle tissue of the eyes. The study demonstrates that the thyroglobulin originated in the thyroid gland. This confirms that the autoimmune reaction that takes place in the thyroid is similar to the autoimmune reaction that takes place in the eyes.

Research published in *Thyroid* in 2005, suggests that an antibody named anti-Gal plays a role in the development of eye problems in Graves' disease. Those people without clinical ophthalmopathy (thyroid eye disease) tended to have lower anti-Gal antibody levels than those with ophthalmopathy. This trend is under further study.

Treating Goitres and Nodules

Goitres and nodules are a common problem in thyroid medicine. Newer studies are changing how doctors manage people with these conditions.

Performing surgery after ethanol injections

One of the newer techniques for eliminating nodules in the thyroid is the injection of ethanol (alcohol) directly into the nodules (refer to Chapter 7). When brand-new, this technique raised the question of whether surgeons would face complications if they had to operate on people receiving ethanol injections. For example, a surgeon might need to operate if the ethanol failed to eliminate a nodule, if a doctor suspected that a nodule was malignant, or if a nodule were compressing a person's trachea.

A study published in *Thyroid* in 2000, reports that surgeons did not encounter any special surgical problems when operating on the thyroids of 13 people who had previously received ethanol injections.

Shrinking goitres

Thyroid hormone is often used to treat goitres in the hope of shrinking the thyroid swelling. Most recent studies show that goitres respond little, if at all, to thyroid hormone.

In a study published in 2001, in the *Journal of Clinical Endocrinology and Metabolism* from the Netherlands, the authors compare thyroid hormone to radioactive iodine in the treatment of goitre.

Using ultrasound to measure the goitre, the study found that people who receive radioactive iodine have, on average, a 44 per cent reduction in goitre size, while those taking thyroid hormone have a reduction of just 1 per cent. Only 1 of 29 patients didn't respond to radioactive iodine, while 16 of 28 had no response to thyroid hormone. Almost half of those receiving radioactive iodine developed hypothyroidism, while 10 of 28 taking thyroid hormone had symptoms of hyperthyroidism. In addition, those on thyroid hormone developed increased bone turnover and a loss of bone mineral density. The conclusion of this study is that radioactive iodine is more effective and better tolerated than thyroid hormone in the treatment of goitres.

Developing New Approaches in Thyroid Cancer

Not surprisingly, much of the research concerning advances in thyroid disease centres around thyroid cancer. The following sections provide you with some of the more provocative and important studies of the last few years. Undoubtedly, many more studies are in the pipeline.

Understanding the impact of radioiodine exposure

More than 15 years after the nuclear disaster in Chernobyl, researchers still follow the children exposed to excessive radioactive iodine. In the *World Journal of Surgery* in 2000, a group of Russian scientists published the results of surgery on 330 children with thyroid cancer after Chernobyl. These cancers tend to develop rapidly after exposure, are more aggressive than typical thyroid cancers, and spread early to distant sites in the body. The children affected are treated with total thyroidectomy (removal of the entire thyroid) then radioactive iodine treatment and suppression of TSH. The authors of the study emphasise that many more cases of thyroid cancer are expected among the children of Chernobyl, and monitoring continues long-term.

Are any environmental factors protective in the situation of radioactive iodine exposure? A study in *Environmental Health* in 2000, looked at people exposed to radioactive iodine in Germany. The study confirms that drinking coffee and eating cruciferous vegetables, such as broccoli, reduces the risk of developing cancer. Broccoli contains substances that help to protect against a number of cancers, but may reduce thyroid function in people lacking in iodine, due to its goitrogen content (see Chapter 12). If a person has a goitre prior to the exposure, or if that person consumes decaffeinated coffee instead of caffeinated, their risk for malignant or benign tumours increases.

The researchers also found that tomato consumption was a risk factor for malignant disease. They suggest that off-season tomatoes coming from areas where the farmers are careless about the use of chemicals may promote the development of thyroid cancer. This news is disappointing since tomatoes are a rich source of the antioxidant carotenoid, lycopene, found in other studies to protect against cancer. Perhaps the message here is to select organically grown produce, especially tomatoes.

Blocking oestrogen slows tumour growth

A source of bewilderment about thyroid cancer is that it occurs around three times more often in women than men. One study suggests the reason may lie with the fact that women make oestrogens as their primary sex hormone, and oestrogen may stimulate thyroid tumour cell growth. One early study published in 1991, found that around 4 per cent of the well-differentiated thyroid cancer biopsies they studied contained oestrogen receptors.

In a more recent study published in the *Journal of Clinical Endocrinology and Metabolism* during 2001, researchers confirmed the presence of oestrogen receptors in cells derived from human goitre nodules and thyroid cancers, but found no difference between the presence of these receptors in males and females. When cells are exposed to an oestrogen, however, the expression rates increase significantly as oestrogen activates a metabolic pathway that leads to much greater growth activity in both malignant and benign thyroid cells. Exposing the cells to a drug that blocks oestrogen action, meant the tumour cells were no longer stimulated.

Women have significantly higher oestrogen levels than males, which may explain why women are more likely to develop these thyroid problems than males.

Predicting thyroid cancer

Can doctors predict the future occurrence of thyroid cancer? In a study from Iceland, the authors present an analysis of blood taken many years before the diagnosis of thyroid cancer in 164 patients. Their study is published in *Acta Oncologica* (2000).

The authors report that levels of thyroglobulin, the chemical that resides in the thyroid, and which is monitored when following people with thyroid cancer, was found in much elevated levels up to 15 years before the diagnosis of thyroid cancer was made. In contrast, no difference was found in the blood levels of TSH or thyroid hormone in those going on to develop thyroid cancer compared to those who do not.

Detecting residual thyroid cancer

Another important recent advance is in the ability to detect thyroid cancer that remains after surgery. Thyroglobulin plays a major role in detecting remaining cancer. Another important tool that is often used is the whole body radioactive iodine scan, which can locate active thyroid tissue. The limitation of the scan is that it can't locate thyroid tissue that isn't making thyroid hormone. Sometimes a thyroglobulin level is high, indicating that active thyroid tissue is present, but the body scan is negative.

A newer type of scan called a PET scan is able to localise thyroid tissue that is not functioning well as thyroid tissue but which is still metabolically active. A study in *Advances in Internal Medicine* in 2001 reviews the successful use of the PET scan for this purpose.

The study points out that the need still exists for new agents that attack these tumour tissues when they are discovered as they don't concentrate radioactive iodine.

If you have thyroid cancer and discover a new growth that does not concentrate radioactive iodine on a thyroid scan, ask your doctor about the possibility of having a PET scan.

Following up thyroid cancer treatment

Do people with treated thyroid cancer need follow-up for life, or does a point arise at which they're considered cured of the disease? The authors of a study in *Annales Chirurgiae et Gynecologica* in 2000, attempt to answer this question.

The researchers followed people for seven months after they have had thyroid surgery then divided them into four groups:

- ✔ **Group I:** Patients with microcancers
- ✔ **Group II:** Patients with no lymph node involvement or metastases, and normal thyroglobulin

> **II-A:** Younger than age 45

> **II-B:** Age 45 or older

- ✔ **Group III:** Patients with cancer with lymph node involvement but a normal thyroglobulin
- ✔ **Group IV:** Patients who have extension of the cancer beyond local lymph nodes or an elevated thyroglobulin

The survival rates for these groups are shown in Table 14-1.

Table 14-1	Survival Rates for Thyroid Cancer Patients	
Study Group	*Length of Time after Surgery*	
	10 Years	*15 Years*
Group I	100 per cent	100 per cent
Group II-A	100 per cent	100 per cent
Group II-B	96 per cent	92 per cent
Group III	100 per cent	100 per cent
Group IV	86 per cent	73 per cent

The latest time a recurrence was found in Groups I and II-A was at 12 years. For Groups II-B, III, and IV, tumours were discovered as late as 16 years after treatment. The study emphasises the importance of carrying out thyroglobulin tests and whole body scanning every 5 years.

Results suggest that people in Groups I and II-A need follow-up for up to 15 years, while other patients need following for 20 years before saying with certainty that the disease is eliminated. If a recurrence occurs, then the patient needs follow-up for another 10 years after treatment, before declaring that he or she is cancer-free.

Knowing what to expect from medullary thyroid cancer

Medullary thyroid cancer (MTC) is different from thyroid cell cancers like follicular or papillary cancer (refer to Chapter 8). MTC arises from the C-cells in the thyroid and is not detectable with radioactive iodine. Cases are divided into hereditary (inherited) MTC and sporadic (not inherited) MTC.

A study from Finland in the *Annales Chiarurgiae et Gynecologica* in 2000, found that sporadic MTC is a more aggressive disease than familial MTC. The debate continues, but it seems that more important predictors of survival are involvement of lymph nodes, distant metastases, and local spread of the cancer in the neck.

Using recombinant TSH to treat thyroid cancer

Scientists can now make TSH in the laboratory by inserting the gene that codes for human TSH into a bacterial culture. The product is known as recombinant TSH and is identical to the TSH normally produced by the pituitary gland. Recombinant TSH is a valuable tool both for the detection and treatment of residual thyroid cancer. Before the development of recombinant TSH, people undergoing testing for residual cancer with a total body scan, were taken off thyroid replacement hormone for four weeks or longer to allow their tissues to become hypothyroid. Going off hormone replacement greatly enhances the uptake of radioactive iodine, allowing for a more accurate scan of thyroid tissue.

This action is of concern as the time off thyroid hormone may allow cancer cells to grow more rapidly. In contrast, recombinant TSH can stimulate uptake and identify cancer recurrences without needing to stop thyroid hormone replacement.

A group in Massachusetts, writing in the *Journal of Clinical Endocrinology and Metabolism* in 2001, explored the dose of recombinant TSH required for optimal effect. They found that a dose of 0.3 milligrams of recombinant TSH produces the maximal increase in thyroglobulin and radioactive iodine uptake. Going higher than 0.3 milligrams doesn't increase the effect of treatment.

Another group from New York shows that using recombinant TSH is just as good as taking people off thyroid medication in stimulating thyroglobulin secretion and radioactive iodine uptake. They conclude that preparing people for a scan with recombinant TSH is equivalent to taking them off thyroid hormone, in terms of diagnostic accuracy. Their work is found in the *European Journal of Endocrinology*, 2001.

Finally, recombinant TSH is useful to stimulate thyroid cancer uptake of radioactive iodine in order to destroy it. In a study published in 2001, in the *European Journal of Endocrinology*, scientists note that the recombinant TSH produces excellent results when used in this way, and was free of side effects other than mild nausea. The thyroid cancer treatment was as effective as with patients who were taken off thyroid hormone therapy prior to treatment. Using recombinant TSH meant patients avoid the discomfort of going without thyroid hormone for weeks.

Testing calcium levels after cancer surgery

During removal of the thyroid gland for thyroid cancer, patients inevitably experience some trauma to the parathyroid glands that lie on the back of the thyroid lobes. Most of the time, these glands recover, but sometimes the trauma results in permanent hypoparathyroidism, which leads to low calcium levels.

In a study published in the *Journal of the European Society of Surgery and Oncology* in 2000, researchers looked at how long it takes people undergoing surgery for thyroid cancer to recover their normal calcium levels, as well as to determine how often treatment is necessary.

The study shows that if a person has just one lobe of the thyroid removed, even though two of the parathyroid glands were not touched, a 10 per cent drop in their calcium level occurred. Just over a third of people undergoing this type of surgery require some calcium treatment because the level falls too low. Their calcium levels returned to normal within one week after surgery and remained normal.

When both sides of the thyroid are operated on, as expected, the greater effect is on the parathyroids and the calcium. Calcium levels decreased by an average of 15 per cent and some people experienced severely low levels early in their recovery. The calcium decline was greater if fewer parathyroid glands were preserved. In 15 per cent of cases, calcium treatment was needed for 2 to 7 days, in 26 per cent for 8 to 180 days, and in 9 per cent for longer than a year. Only 1 patient out of 82 required permanent treatment for low calcium after a single thyroid surgery on both sides, while one of four who had several thyroid surgeries needed permanent calcium treatment.

Tackling Iodine Deficiency Disease

The number of people affected by iodine deficiency disease is high (refer to Chapter 12) and lots of research is going on in this area. This section describes the more important recent studies on iodine deficiency disease.

Recognising the importance of selenium

Selenium is a trace element that plays a role in thyroid hormone production, as it forms part of a seleno-enzyme responsible for converting T4 into T3. Until recently, researchers believed that selenium deficiency alone does not cause hypothyroidism and that selenium deficiency only contributes to the disease when iodine deficiency exists. However, a study from the journal *Biological Trace Element Research* in 2000, describes three girls with hypothyroidism due to lack of selenium alone. When given replacement selenium, all returned to normal thyroid function. This study is the first description of hypothyroidism due to lack of selenium alone.

Using iodised oil for goitres

Iodised oil injection is commonly used to treat iodine deficiency and prevent goitre formation in areas of the world where iodine deficiency persists (refer to Chapter 12). The authors of a study in *Medicine* in 2001, looked at potential problems associated with Lipiodol – a type of iodised oil. The study found that, when Lipiodol is given to someone who already has a multinodular goitre, the person sometimes becomes hyperthyroid. The hyperthyroidism tends to be mild and doesn't last long, however. If given to a pregnant woman, the iodine sometimes entered the bloodstream of the foetus but did not cause a problem there.

The study confirms that using iodised oil for the replacement of iodine is a safe, cheap, and effective way to treat this deficiency.

Increasing the intelligence of babies born to hypothyroid mothers

Babies born to hypothyroid mothers tend to have reduced intelligence. A study from Taiwan, published in the *Journal of the Formosan Medical Association* in 2001, looked at the level of intelligence of 62 babies of hypothyroid mothers and sought an early screening to avoid disability. They found that the level of T4 at the time of diagnosis was a good predictor of the future intelligence of the baby. By measuring T4 at birth and giving replacement thyroid hormone, they significantly improved the outlook for these babies in terms of their intelligence.

As you can see, just about every aspect of thyroid disease is being studied, with articles in every medical journal. If you have a particular problem that concerns you or a loved one, don't hesitate to use the enormous, free resources at your disposal. Go to the Pub Med Web page, `www.ncbi.nlm.nih.gov/PubMed`, or check out your local bookstore and library. And be sure to utilise the references you find in Appendix B of this book.

Chapter 15

Living with Thyroid Problems: Diet and Exercise

· ·

In This Chapter

▶ Working to assure your best nutrition

▶ Evaluating your thyroid and weight loss

▶ Remembering the importance of iodine

▶ Using exercise to maintain thyroid and body health

▶ Understanding leptin and your thyroid

· ·

*Y*our thyroid gland functions at its best if it finds itself in a healthy body whose tissues receive the right nutrients and whose muscles and bones are strengthened by an appropriate level of exercise. In this chapter we give you a guide on how to easily determine your ideal weight for your height, and discusses some basic ideas about diet and exercise.

Guaranteeing Your Best Nutrition

Two friends run into each other, and the first friend asks how the second one feels. The second friend answers, 'Lousy, I've got arthritis, a bad back, I'm always tense, I have insomnia. Miserable, I'm miserable.' 'And what kind of work are you doing?' the first friend asks. 'The same thing – I'm still selling health foods.'

This story is good for a chuckle, but the truth is that your diet and lifestyle habits, such as drinking and smoking, have more influence on your health than all the diseases in a textbook of medicine.

A number of organisations have published healthy eating guidelines to help you follow the optimum, healthy diet. These messages include suggestions such as:

✔ Enjoy your food

✔ Eat as wide a variety of foods as possible

✔ Eat the right amount to maintain a healthy weight

✔ Eat more fruit and vegetables to ensure you get sufficient vitamins and minerals in your diet – five or more servings of fruit and vegetables per day is ideal

✔ Eat plenty of wholegrain foods rich in fibre

✔ Consider the overall balance of fats in your diet and don't eat too much of any

✔ Eat at least two portions of fish, including one of oily fish per week

✔ Switch to reduced-fat spreads and dairy products from full-fat ones

✔ Eat more monounsaturated fats (for example, olive oil)

✔ Use salt and sugar in moderation

✔ Consume alcoholic beverages, if you do so, in moderation

Foods aren't really good or bad for you – getting a healthy balance is what counts. Keep fatty, sugary foods as occasional treats because banning foods altogether can make you fancy them even more.

Maintaining a Healthy Weight

If you go online and check out a message board about thyroid disease, you'll probably find that lots of people have lots of questions about how the thyroid affects weight gain and loss. This section helps set the record straight. Maintaining a healthy weight is important to help reduce your risk of a number of health problems including:

✔ Diabetes

✔ High blood pressure

✔ Abnormal blood cholesterol levels

✔ Hardening and furring up of the arteries

✔ Coronary heart disease and stroke

Calculating your body mass index

Your body fat stores are usually estimated using the Body Mass Index (BMI). This figure is calculated by dividing your weight in kilograms by your height in metres squared:

BMI = Weight (Kg) ÷ Height (m) ÷ Height (m)

This calculation gives you a figure that is interpreted as follows:

< 20	**Underweight**
20–25	**Healthy weight**
25–30	**Overweight**
30–40	**Obese**
> 40	**Severe obesity**

For example, if your height is 5 feet 7 inches (1.7 metres), and your weight is 12 stone (76 kilograms) your BMI is calculated as 76 divided by 1.7, then divided by 1.7 again = 26.29, which means you're slightly overweight.

As this calculation is too complicated for someone with a life to perform, Table 15-1 makes it easy for you. This table shows the healthy weight range for your height (for adults), based on a BMI of $20 - 25$ kg/M^2. If, for example, someone is 5 feet 7 inches (1.7 metres) and they weigh 12 stone (76 kilograms), they are above their ideal weight range of between 9 stone 1 pound and 11 stone 4 pounds (58–72 kilograms). If your weight falls above the range given for your height, try to lose weight slowly and steadily until you reach the healthy range for your height.

You need to be aware that this calculation is meant as a broad guide only, and should not replace a visit to your doctor for advice on how to safely lose weight. The BMI doesn't take into account your gender or body type, for example, if you're a very muscular male this fact isn't reflected in the calculation as muscle weighs heavier than fat.

Table 15-1	Body Mass Index Healthy Weight Range in Relation to Height	
Height (Metres/Feet)	*Weight*	*(Kilograms/Stones)*
1.47 4'10"	43–54	6st 11–8st 7lb
1.50 4'11"	45–56	7st 1–8st 11lb

(continued)

Table 15-1 *(continued)*

Height (Metres/Feet)	Weight	(Kilograms/Stones)
1.52 5ft	46–58	7st 3–9st 2lb
1.55 5'1"	48–60	7st 8–9st 7lb
1.57 5'2"	49–62	7st 10–9st 11lb
1.60 5'3"	51–64	8st–10st 1lb
1.63 5'4"	53–66	8st 5–10st 6lb
1.65 5'5"	54–68	8st 7–10st 10lb
1.68 5'6"	56–70	8st 12–11st
1.70 5'7"	58–72	9st 1–11st 4
1.73 5'8"	60–75	9st 6–11st 10
1.75 5'9"	61–76	9st 9–12st
1.78 5'10"	63–79	9st 13–12st 6
1.80 5'11"	65–81	10st 3–12st 9
1.83 6 ft	67–83	10st 7–13st 1
1.85 6'1"	69–85	10st 11–13st 5
1.88 6'2"	71–88	11st 2–13st 12
1.90 6'3"	72–90	11st 5–14st 2
1.93 6'4"	75–93	11st 10–14st 8

Measuring your waist size

When you are overweight, the place where you store your excess weight is important. If you store excess fat round your middle (apple-shaped), you're twice as likely to develop coronary heart disease as someone storing excess fat around their hips (pear-shaped). To work out if you are apple-shaped, measure your waist and hip in centimetres using a non-stretchable tape measure. Divide your waist measurement by your hip measurement to get your waist to hip ratio.

For example, if your waist is 88 centimetres, and your hips are 100 centimetres, then your waist to hip ratio is 88/100 = 0.88.

A waist/hip ratio greater than 0.85 is apple-shaped for women, while a ratio greater than 0.95 is apple-shaped for men.

In fact, waist size alone is a good indicator of health. Research suggests that men with a waist circumference larger than 102 centimetres and women with a waist circumference larger than 88 centimetres are more likely to have shortness of breath, high blood pressure, high cholesterol levels, and diabetes than those with slimmer waistlines. Slight waist reductions of just 5–10 centimetres can significantly reduce your risk of a heart attack.

Losing excess weight

The best way to lose weight permanently is to change your eating habits, so you eat more healthily without feeling as if you're actually on a diet. Look on losing weight as a healthy eating plan for the rest of your life, rather than a temporary slimming phase.

Importantly, to lose weight you also need to increase your level of physical activity. Exercise burns off excess calories and boosts your metabolic rate as well as improving the fitness of your heart and lungs. Try to exercise for at least 30 minutes on five days per week. Once you are fit, aim to do more. Start off slowly if you are unfit, and build up to exercise briskly enough to work up a light sweat and make yourself slightly breathless. Try these effective forms of exercise:

- ✔ Brisk walking
- ✔ Cycling
- ✔ Swimming
- ✔ Dancing
- ✔ Vigorous housework
- ✔ Gardening

Don't set yourself unrealistic targets. At first, just aim to stop your weight increasing and prevent the downhill spiral. Then look at how you can slowly lose the pounds – just one or two pounds per week soon adds up to a significant weight loss over the coming months.

Selecting a variety of foods

You've probably heard the phrase 'eat a balanced diet' many times, but what exactly does that mean? Eating a balanced diet just means eating enough of the right sorts of foods, in the right amounts, to provide all the energy, carbohydrate, protein, fat, vitamins, and minerals you need on a daily basis. A healthy, balanced diet gives you:

✔ Enough energy to fuel your level of physical activity and maintain a healthy weight

✔ Enough protein for tissue repair, regeneration, and rejuvenation

✔ Enough essential fatty acids (omega-3) that your body is unable to produce itself

✔ At least the recommended daily amount of vitamins and minerals

✔ Enough fluid to maintain a normal water balance

Different people need different amounts of foods depending on their level of physical activity – both at work and leisure – their height, weight, age, and the metabolism they have inherited. In general, however, most people benefit from eating:

✔ More starchy (complex or unrefined) carbohydrates, such as wholegrain cereals

✔ More fresh fruit and vegetables

✔ More unsalted nuts and seeds

✔ More fish, especially oily fish

✔ Less fat, especially saturated fat

✔ Less processed, ready-made products

Most people obtain more than enough protein from their diet, and cutting back on fatty foods and those that are protein-rich helps to make room for more fruit and vegetables.

The food proportions that help to make up a balanced diet are illustrated on a plate diagram.

As you can see in Figure 15-1, all types of foods are included – even chocolate and biscuits. There are no such things as 'good' or 'bad' foods in a healthy, balanced diet as long as you go easy on sugary, fatty foods and do not eat them in excess. The five main food groups included in the plate diagram are:

✔ **Fruit and vegetables:** Fresh, frozen, and canned; pure juices and dried fruits. Try to eat at least five portions of fruit and veg a day. As a rough guide, a portion is:

　• 1 small glass of fruit juice

　• 2 tablespoons of vegetables

　• 1 piece of fresh fruit

　• Small handful of fruits, such as grapes or strawberries

　• Small bowl of salad

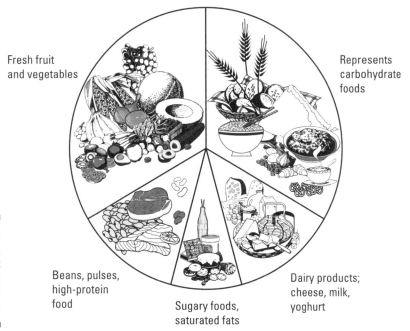

Fresh fruit and vegetables

Represents carbohydrate foods

Beans, pulses, high-protein food

Sugary foods, saturated fats

Dairy products; cheese, milk, yoghurt

Figure 15-1: Food types, and the part they play in a balanced diet.

✔ **Lean meat, poultry, fish, and vegetarian alternatives:** Altogether, you need to eat two or three servings of these protein-rich foods per day, where one serving counts as:

- 60–90 grams (2–3 ounces) of meat, poultry, or oily fish

- Small can of beans

- 240 grams (8 ounces) of cooked pulses

- 120 grams (4 ounces) of fish

- 1 egg (not fried)

Try to have fish twice a week, including one portion of oily fish (for example, salmon, herring, mackerel, sardines, and pilchards). Alternative sources of protein are pulses, nuts, seeds, and soya products.

✔ **Milk and dairy foods:** Try to select low-fat versions such as semi-skimmed or skimmed milk, and lower fat cheeses such as Gouda, Edam, or cottage cheese. Aim to eat 2–3 measures of these a day, where a measure is:

- 200 millilitres (one-third of a pint) of semi-skimmed/skimmed milk

- 30 grams (1 ounce) of cheese

- 1 small pot of yoghurt

- 120 grams (4 ounces) of cottage cheese

✔ **Bread, cereals, and potatoes:** This group includes savoury crackers, noodles, oats, chapattis, pasta, and rice. You can eat 5–14 measures of these foods per day, depending on your energy needs (manual workers need more than office workers, for example). A measure is:

- 1 slice of bread

- 5 tablespoons of breakfast cereal

- 2 tablespoons of cooked rice, pasta, or noodles

- 2 egg-sized potatoes

✔ **Fatty and sugary foods:** Includes margarine and butter, cooking oils and sugar. In a healthy balanced diet, these foods are used in moderation only, so watch your intake of fried foods, crisps, biscuits, and high-fat, high-sugar snacks. Most people eat far too many of these foods, so cut right back on them and use low-fat, low-sugar products where possible.

Taking vital vitamins

Although vitamins are only needed in tiny amounts, they are essential for health. Vitamins are involved in energy-producing chemical reactions in your body and must come from your diet as your body cannot make them. The various vitamins, their function, and their sources in food include the following:

✔ **Vitamin A:** Used for vision and growth of bone and teeth, is found in liver, carrots, and spinach.

✔ **Vitamin B1:** Used for digestion and nervous system function, comes from wholegrain cereals, peas, and nuts.

✔ **Vitamin B2:** Helps to release energy and maintain the skin and eyes, comes from liver, milk, eggs, and green leafy vegetables.

✔ **Vitamin B3:** Used for maintenance of the skin and nerves, comes from chicken, salmon, and peanuts.

✔ **Vitamin B6:** Needed to make red blood cells and to release energy from the energy sources. It comes from meat, fish, poultry, and peanuts.

✔ **Vitamin B12:** Essential for the nervous system and red blood cells. It's found in all foods coming from animals, including meat and milk; a person who eats nothing but vegetables doesn't get this vitamin.

✔ **Vitamin C:** Helps with healing and prevention of infections and is found in citrus fruits, strawberries, and broccoli.

✔ **Vitamin D:** Required for the absorption of dietary calcium in the gut and comes in milk, fish, and the yolk of eggs. Fortunately, this is a vitamin that can be made by the body when the skin is exposed to sunlight.

✔ **Vitamin E:** Functions include the prevention of cholesterol build-up and production of red blood cells and muscles. You get it in vegetable oils, peas, and nuts.

✔ **Vitamin K:** Essential for clotting of the blood so that you don't continue to bleed when you are cut. It's found in broccoli and green leafy vegetables.

✔ **Folic acid:** Needed to produce red blood cells and protein. It's found in green leafy vegetables, oranges, and peanuts.

Maintaining your minerals

The mineral content of your food depends on the mineral content of the soil in which plants are grown and animals are reared. Minerals are divided into *major minerals*, which are present in relatively large amounts in the body, and *trace elements* that are essential but present in only tiny amounts.

The major minerals consist of the following:

✔ **Calcium:** For strong bones and teeth, for blood clotting, and for muscle function, found in dairy products, almonds, broccoli, and other green leafy vegetables.

✔ **Magnesium:** For nerve and muscle function, found in milk, seafood, bananas, and green leafy vegetables.

✔ **Phosphorus:** For the bones and teeth, comes from milk, hamburger, and cheese.

The trace elements include:

✔ **Chromium:** Needed for production of glucose tolerance factor, which interacts with insulin hormone to control the way cells take up glucose. Found in organ meats, mushrooms, and broccoli.

✔ **Iodine:** The key mineral for the production of thyroid hormones, which is found in seafood and iodised salt and bread.

✔ **Iron:** For red blood cell haemoglobin, comes from meat, poultry, fish, and raisins.

✔ **Selenium:** Also used in enzymes that affect thyroid hormones, found in seafood and wholegrains.

✔ **Zinc:** Needed in the production of insulin and found in red meat, shellfish, and eggs.

Now you know what these nutrients are, what they do, and where they can be found. No discussion of proper nutrition could leave out a discussion of fats, so keep reading.

Choosing your fats wisely

Nutritionists advise limiting your fat intake to no more than 30 per cent of your total daily calories, while limiting your intake of saturated fat to no more than one third of that amount, that is, no more than 10 per cent of your total daily calories.

You can keep your fats down by looking for low-fat foods, which are plentiful in the supermarkets these days. Just remember not to substitute foods rich in carbohydrates. Food labels can tell you what you need to know about the energy sources in the food as well as the amounts of the vitamins and minerals.

When checking labels for fat content, a good general rule is that, per 100 grams food (or per serving if a serving is less than 100 grams):

- ✔ **3 grams** of total fat or less is **a little** fat
- ✔ **20 grams** of total fat or more is **a lot** of fat

While for saturated fats:

- ✔ **1 gram** of saturated fat or less is **a little** saturated fat
- ✔ **5 grams** of saturated fat or more is **a lot** of saturated fat

Checking out your cholesterol

The fat that most people think about is *cholesterol*. Ask your doctor to check your cholesterol level if you don't know it yet. The average Total Cholesterol level for adults aged 35–64 years is currently 6.1 mmol/L (millimoles per litre), significantly higher than the target healthy Total Cholesterol level of less than 5 mmol/L (millimoles per litre). However, you have two types of cholesterol in your circulation:

- ✔ Low-density lipoprotein (LDL) cholesterol – often referred to as 'bad cholesterol' as high levels are linked with hardening and furring up of artery walls, high blood pressure, and coronary heart disease.

- ✔ High-density lipoprotein (HDL) cholesterol – usually referred to as 'good cholesterol' as it helps to protect against heart disease by transporting LDL-cholesterol away from the arteries and back to the liver for processing.

Although knowing your total cholesterol level is useful, the relative level of LDL-cholesterol and HDL-cholesterol is more important. This ratio is closely linked with your future risk of heart attack and stroke, which together account for as many as 245,000 deaths each year in the United Kingdom.

An ideal LDL-cholesterol level is less than 3 mmol/L (millimoles per litre), while an ideal HDL-cholesterol level is greater than 1 mmol/L (millimoles per litre).

You can do a simple calculation to see whether your level of cholesterol is potentially harmful. Divide your total cholesterol level (for example, 6) with your HDL cholesterol level (for example 1) and if the result is less than 4.5, you have a low risk of having a heart attack. The higher that number, the greater you're at risk. Obviously, other factors such as your blood pressure, age, gender, and glucose levels also play a role, but this calculation is useful to see whether or not you need to worry about your cholesterol levels.

You can do something to raise your HDL or 'good' cholesterol. The best way is exercise. The more you do (within reason), the higher your HDL and the lower your risk of having a heart attack.

High cholesterol is also a well-known effect of hypothyroidism. Moreover, high cholesterol is not only associated with coronary heart disease and heart attacks, but with peripheral vascular disease (leading to blocked blood flow to the legs) and cerebral artery disease, which can lead to strokes.

The number of people with high cholesterol is far greater than the number of people who have hypothyroidism. Most abnormalities in cholesterol are due to excessive fat in the diet and lack of exercise.

However, there are undoubtedly many cases of undiagnosed hypothyroidism that do result in high cholesterol. Studies show that more than 10 per cent of people with high cholesterol (levels over 5 mmol/L) have hypothyroidism. Most people with high cholesterol are not tested for hypothyroidism, and most people don't know that hypothyroidism and high cholesterol have a connection in the first place.

When someone with high cholesterol is diagnosed with hypothyroidism, the treatment is, of course, thyroid hormone. The results are often pretty dramatic, however, with cholesterol levels falling as much as 30–40 per cent when someone with hypothyroidism takes thyroid hormone. However, this is not always true for people with subclinical hypothyroidism, where they have an elevated TSH level but a normal free T4.

The explanation for the increase in cholesterol in hypothyroidism is that the breakdown of cholesterol declines with hypothyroidism just as the metabolism of everything else in the body declines. However, the production of cholesterol remains the same, leading to a rise in the blood cholesterol.

If your cholesterol is elevated above 5 mmol/L (millimoles per litre), ask your doctor to check your thyroid function.

Moderating your sugar intake

Most people are aware that excess sugar is bad for your health. The many reasons for this include:

- Sugary foods promote tooth decay.

- Sugary foods often contain few essential nutrients and replace those foods that have these nutrients.

- Sugary foods are the source of many calories. They are often eaten in an effort to avoid fatty foods, but you still end up with too many calories.

- Excess sugar increases insulin secretion, which lowers blood glucose levels. Sugar swings can cause tiredness and lethargy.

- A high-sugar diet increases the risk of developing Type 2 diabetes

You can avoid these problems if you keep to small, infrequent portions of sugary foods such as pies, cakes, candies, and biscuits. Substituting fruit for these sugary foods reduces sugar intake, provides a certain amount of sweetness for your sweet tooth, and provides other important nutrients at the same time.

The biggest offender when it comes to lots of sugar with no nutrition is sugar-based fizzy drinks. Unless you choose diet soda, prepared with non-caloric sweeteners, the typical bottle of soda gives you a huge amount of sugar and nothing else. Even the flavoured fruit sodas are loaded with sugar. Do yourself a favour and switch to water with lemon or lime or the diet sodas that contain no sugar. Always read the label first before selecting a fizzy drink.

Sifting the salt

Guidelines regarding salt intake are designed to help protect you from developing high blood pressure. The recommended amount of salt is no more than a teaspoon, or 6 grams, daily. Most people eat twice as much as that, or more. One problem is that food manufacturers typically add a lot of salt to their foods. To help avoid this, check labels and choose low-salt foods. A good rule of thumb is that, per 100 grams food (or per serving if a serving is less than 100 grams):

- ✔ **0.5 grams** sodium or more is **a lot** of sodium

- ✔ **0.1 grams** sodium or less is **a little** sodium

When you read food labels, multiply those giving salt content as 'sodium' by 2.5 to give table salt content. For example, a serving of soup containing 0.4 grams sodium contains 1 gram salt (sodium chloride).

Another problem is that people are too used to picking up the salt shaker and heavily spraying their food with salt. The result is food that tastes like salt and not much else. Try your food without salt for a change. At first it tastes bland, but you soon begin to notice the subtle flavours of the food coming through. Using black pepper, herbs, and lime juice all help give food more flavour while waiting for your taste buds to readjust.

Most recipes, especially in older cookbooks, recommend more salt than is necessary for proper preparation of the food. Try reducing the salt in the recipe by half – or leaving it out altogether (except perhaps for bread). In most cases, the food cooks just as well and the taste is even superior. If you don't tell your family about reducing the salt, chances are they'll never notice.

In many countries, iodised salt is the major source of iodine (refer to Chapter 12). That teaspoon of salt a day contains twice as much iodine as you need each day, so you can reduce your salt intake to a half teaspoon and still know you're getting enough salt. If you eat one piece of bread, it contains just about your daily requirement of iodine. You do not need to eat excess salt to assure yourself of getting enough iodine.

Drinking alcohol in moderation

If you consume more than one or two drinks of alcohol a day or more than ten in a week, do your best to reduce those amounts. Like cigarettes, alcohol damages your body in many ways (although small amounts are beneficial). Excess alcohol consumption

- ✔ Raises your blood pressure

- ✔ Increases your risk of a heart attack

- ✔ Damages your liver

- ✔ Promotes certain cancers

Drinking to excess provides no nutrition and often causes you to eat less of the foods you need for good nutrition. Severe alcoholism results in:

✔ Damage to the nervous system

✔ Vitamin deficiency diseases

✔ Anaemia

✔ Skin damage

Alcohol also destroys families. When one or more members of a family are alcoholic, the incidence of divorce, accidents, suicide, loss of employment, and disease within that family is much greater than in families that do not have an alcoholic member. Alcoholism can also lead to impotency, making sexual relations impossible.

Keep in mind that alcohol in moderation can raise the level of HDL or 'good' cholesterol in your body. Alcohol is also a pleasant part of a meal and a key element in certain social scenes. Clearly, alcohol is not going to go away, but do use it wisely.

Going Organic

To protect yourself from chemicals sprayed on foods as they are grown and chemicals present in the soil that fruits and vegetables are grown in, wash all fruits and vegetables before eating them, and peel root vegetables, such as carrots. Obviously, this action doesn't eliminate chemicals inside the food, and some people choose to pay a little extra and buy organic crops. Organically grown produce is cultivated using traditional methods and many people find they taste better as they are not grown for uniformity of size, shape, and colour above flavour. They are often more nutritious, too, with a higher content of vitamins and minerals, and less water.

Thinking about food safety

Properly refrigerating foods that spoil quickly, such as meat, fish, and poultry, is essential. Keeping your fridge temperature below 5 degrees C (and freezer temperature below –18 degrees C) is ideal. Keep your hands clean when you handle these foods. And make sure that cutting boards and knives are cleaned well after you use them for cutting raw meats. Keep pets away from food preparation areas, and cover food to help keep flies at bay. The use of a mild bleach solution to cleanse cutting boards and kitchen surfaces is a good idea. Always cook foods thoroughly. After you cook food, if you want to save it for a later time, keep it in the refrigerator. Leaving it at room temperature allows bacteria to grow and produces toxins that can cause food poisoning even if the food is thoroughly reheated to piping hot.

Clarifying the Thyroid–Weight Connection

Certain misconceptions exist about how your thyroid reacts to weight loss, and how your weight reacts to a change in your thyroid function. This section helps to dispel these misconceptions as it explains how your thyroid and your weight really interact.

Does my metabolism slow when I lose weight?

People who lose weight on a diet often regain the weight after a time. You may have heard that the reason you can't keep weight off is because your thyroid and metabolism slow down after you've lost some pounds, so weight comes back on more easily. This reasoning implies that your body establishes a 'set point' weight and tries to maintain it through changing your thyroid function and your metabolism whenever you move away from that weight. The idea is that if you lose weight, your metabolic rate falls because your thyroid function declines. Researchers have studied this idea to determine its validity.

In a study in the *American Journal of Clinical Nutrition*, 2000, researchers tested thyroid function and metabolic rates for 24 overweight women in the process of losing weight. When actively losing weight, the women's resting metabolic rates and free T3 hormone levels declined. But after reaching their normal weight, their free T3 levels and resting metabolic rate remained normal. This study contradicts the idea of a 'set point' weight.

If you are having trouble keeping off the weight you lose and your thyroid is functioning normally, this study shows that your thyroid is not to blame. You may want to take a closer look at your exercise and eating habits instead.

If I'm treated for hyperthyroidism, am I doomed to gain weight?

Many people who are treated for hyperthyroidism with radioactive iodine complain that they cannot lose weight after they become hypothyroid and are placed on thyroid hormone replacement. If this describes your situation, you should consider a number of possible explanations:

✔ Perhaps you're not taking enough thyroid hormones to replace your deficit. Importantly, check that your thyroid-stimulating hormone (TSH) is in the normal range, and ideally less than 2.5.

✔ You may need to take T3 hormone replacement as well as T4, even if your TSH is normal (refer to Chapter 4), although this treatment is controversial in the United Kingdom.

✔ Perhaps you're eating foods that interfere with thyroid hormone absorption, such as soy protein, around the time you take the thyroid hormone tablet.

Then again, it's possible that none of the above can explain your weight gain. A study in the *Journal of the American College of Nutrition* in 1999, attempted to address this issue. The authors studied 10 people treated with radioactive iodine for hyperthyroidism. The researchers looked at the participants' total food energy intake; their T4, T3, and TSH levels; and their height and weight at the time of treatment and at 1, 2, 3, 6, and 12 months afterwards.

The participants' thyroid hormone levels declined in the first months of treatment but increased later. Even when thyroid hormone levels increased, the participants continued to gain weight.

Interestingly, the average weight of the participants before the development of hyperthyroidism was about 170 pounds; at the time of treatment, 148 pounds; and after a year, about 168 pounds. Their final average weight was actually lower than their average weight before hyperthyroidism developed. The study concludes that weight gain after treatment of hyperthyroidism is initially due to a fall in the metabolic rate that accompanies the drop in thyroid hormone but later is due to food intake or lifestyle choices.

Another study, in the *Journal of Clinical Endocrinology and Metabolism* in 1998, showed where weight gain occurs in the body when hyperthyroidism is treated. Most of the weight gain in the first three months occurs as fat in the waist area and in muscle tissue, whereas weight gain later on is in the fat under the skin. This study shows very clearly that the weight loss occurring before treatment for hyperthyroidism is loss of lean tissue, the muscle mass. (Therefore, further proof that using excess thyroid hormone for weight loss leads to loss of muscle.)

Many people treated for hyperthyroidism gain more weight than they want to after treatment. In most cases, this occurs either because their thyroid hormone levels are not in the ideal range, or because they do not alter their eating and exercise habits after treatment. If you're in this situation, keep in mind that you probably increased your food intake and decreased your activity level when hyperthyroid. You need to make lifestyle adjustments after treatment in order to bring your body back to its healthy weight.

The thyroid and coeliac condition

Coeliac condition is an autoimmune disease of the small intestine that results in poor absorption of fat, protein, carbohydrates, iron, and vitamins A, D, and K. The consequences of coeliac condition are diarrhoea, osteomalacia (poorly mineralised bone), signs of vitamin deficiency, and anaemia. Studies show that as high as 21 per cent of people with coeliac condition also have autoimmune hypothyroidism, and 3 per cent of people with thyroid disease have coeliac condition.

The treatment for coeliac condition is to remove gluten from the diet. Gluten is found in wheat, barley, and rye, and as a filler in many prepared foods and medications. When gluten is removed from the diet, not only does coeliac condition disappear, but the thyroid disease is cured as well.

A study in the American Journal of Gastro-enterology in March 2001, found that out of 241 people with coeliac condition, 31 (13 per cent) also had hypothyroidism. Of the 31, 29 had sub-clinical hypothyroidism with an elevation in TSH but a normal T4. After avoiding gluten in their diet for a year, the coeliac condition was cured, and the thyroid abnormalities disappeared in all of them as well.

Thyroid disease is so commonly associated with coeliac condition that everyone suffering from it should have a thyroid function test. If present, both the coeliac condition and the thyroid disorder may respond to gluten withdrawal.

Considering Iodine in Your Diet

Because iodine is a key element of thyroid hormones, iodine is a necessary part of your everyday diet (refer to Chapter 3). However, the consequences of not having enough iodine are dramatic and devastating to your health. (Refer to Chapter 12 for the vastness of the problem in many countries and why this deficiency occurs.) This section shows you how to include iodine in your daily diet if you don't eat animal products, and the occasions when you shouldn't take too much of it.

Getting enough iodine in a vegetarian diet

Vegetarians, and especially vegans, do not eat key foods that contain iodine, such as fish, seafood, eggs, meat, and milk. You need to have sufficient iodine in your diet for good thyroid health. A study of vegetarians published in the *British Journal of Medicine* in December 1998, found that 63 per cent of the females and 36 per cent of the males had inadequate iodine intake.

If you follow a vegetarian diet, consider taking iodised salt or iodine supplements. A slice or two of bread also helps to take care of your iodine needs as a vegetarian.

Avoiding iodine before thyroid studies

The results of thyroid uptake studies are more valuable if you avoid foods that contain iodine for a time before the test. The purpose of most such studies is to determine the size and shape of your thyroid and whether or not a given abnormality of the thyroid takes up iodine.

If you are having tests for hyperthyroidism, you don't need to avoid iodine. In fact, avoiding iodine may confuse the diagnosis because the test is looking for abnormally high uptake of iodine, and you do not want to artificially enhance the test results by following a low-iodine diet.

If you're having a thyroid scan for reasons other than hyperthyroidism, follow a low-iodine diet for several days:

✔ Use only non-iodised salt

✔ Avoid milk and milk products

✔ Avoid commercial vitamin preparations unless they definitely do not contain iodine

✔ Steer clear of eggs

✔ Don't eat seafood, fish, shellfish, seaweed, and kelp

✔ Avoid cured and corned foods (for example, ham, smoked fish, and tinned corned beef)

✔ Don't use bread products made with iodine dough conditioners

✔ Avoid foods that contain Red Dye # 3, chocolate, molasses, and soy

Exercising for Your Thyroid

If tests show that you have normal thyroid function, you can exercise as much as you want. Just ensure that you listen to your body and slow down if you feel you're overextending yourself. The best form of activity is aerobic exercise, in which your heart is forced to beat faster, to keep your circulation healthy and your body fat under control. Also aim to do some strength training to retain and build muscle.

If tests show that your thyroid function is not yet within the normal range, you need to take special considerations regarding exercise, which are discussed in this section.

Recognising the natural consequences of ageing

Don't confuse the natural effects of ageing with the consequences of having thyroid disease. As you get older, your ability to do aerobic exercise is going to decrease, as is your strength. If you go to the gym for the first time in years and find you can't last as long on the treadmill as you used to, chances are that your thyroid isn't the culprit.

Your ability to take in oxygen is a measure of your physical condition. Your oxygen uptake peaks around the age of 25, and after that, it steadily declines no matter what you do to prevent it. Your strength also seems to peak around the same time, but it remains more or less the same until around age 40, when it starts to decline steadily. We lose about 25 per cent of our maximum strength by age 65. We also lose flexibility with ageing – our tendons, ligaments, and joint capsules become stiffer.

You have almost certainly heard the old saying, 'You're only young once.' Unfortunately: It's true.

At any age, exercise can maximise your strength, your stamina, and your flexibility, however. To achieve this benefit, aim for at least 30 minutes exercise, at least 5 times a week, and preferably every day.

Working out with hypothyroidism

When you have an underactive thyroid, your ability to exercise is limited by the fatigue that accompanies this condition. After you have begun taking the proper replacement dose of thyroid hormone, you can usually start to exercise normally. If you still can't exercise because of fatigue, consider the two most common reasons:

- ✔ Perhaps you're not receiving sufficient thyroid hormone so your TSH is between 0.5 and 2.5 mU/ml (microunits per millilitre). If your symptoms linger even after taking the hormone replacement, don't settle for a TSH of 3 mU/ml or higher.
- ✔ You may need to take T3 hormone in addition to T4 to fully replace your missing thyroid function (although this treatment is controversial in the United Kingdom).

Hypothyroidism does affect the functioning of your heart, which is often apparent during exercise. If you're receiving treatment with thyroid hormone, your heart function should return to normal (assuming that you don't have any other heart conditions).

Heart function during exercise is often a greater issue for people with subclinical hypothyroidism (where your TSH is elevated but your free T4 is normal), because this condition is often not treated with thyroid hormone. (Refer to Chapter 14 for a detailed discussion of the debate over treatment.) Subclinical hypothyroidism is associated with mild abnormalities in the heart, which are not measurable when you are resting but are detected when you exercise. The normal ability of your heart to adapt to effort is diminished in subclinical hypothyroidism. Subclinical hypothyroidism also results in a rise in the form of cholesterol that leads to heart attacks and a fall in the form that is protective against heart attacks. Some thyroid specialists believe that these subtle changes are reason enough to treat subclinical hypothyroidism with thyroid hormone.

The muscles of a person with subclinical hypothyroidism show abnormal energy metabolism that leads to early fatigue; this is also corrected with thyroid hormone. The ability of blood vessels to open up to allow more blood flow is also impaired. This fact is further evidence of the need for treatment, particularly before the condition worsens.

Exercising with hyperthyroidism

If you have hyperthyroidism, your heart rate and the amount of blood pumped per heartbeat are both elevated when you are resting, but they do not respond to exercise in a normal fashion. After normal thyroid function is achieved through treatment, these abnormalities disappear.

Careful study of the hearts of people with hyperthyroidism shows that their resting heart rates are abnormally high, as are the frequent occurrences of abnormal heart rhythms. The size of the heart is increased as a result of abnormal thickening of the heart muscle.

With exercise, the hyperthyroid heart cannot increase its workload in the same way as a normal heart. The result is that someone with hyperthyroidism cannot exercise as long as he or she used to, and his or her peak level of exercise is reduced. This fact is true even in subclinical hyperthyroidism, where the TSH is suppressed below the normal range but the free T4 remains normal. When the beta-blocker drug propranolol is given to slow the heart rate, the person often feels an improvement in exercise capacity (although one of the possible side effects of beta-blockers is fatigue).

An older person with hyperthyroidism needs to be especially careful with exercise because older people have an increased risk of heart failure, and may experience abnormal heart rhythms (which may not improve even when the hyperthyroidism is brought under control). Chest pain can get worse as hyperthyroidism continues.

Not only heart muscle but also skeletal (arm, leg, and trunk) muscles are abnormal in hyperthyroidism. Hyperthyroid skeletal muscle requires more energy to perform the same amount of work as healthy muscle. As a result, the muscle is fatigued much earlier.

Meeting your minimal exercise needs

While you are recovering from hypothyroidism or hyperthyroidism, you often can't do much exercise and certainly not the amount necessary for good health. After you are cured, however, you want to get up to speed.

You want to do two types of exercise:

- ✔ **Aerobic exercise:** To improve heart and lung function, and raise your healthy HDL-cholesterol level.
- ✔ **Anaerobic exercise:** To strengthen muscles and increase stamina.

Any exercise that gets your heart beating faster for a sustained period is aerobic exercise. Doctors used to recommend a formula for determining the ideal heart rate during exercise: Subtract your age from 220, and your ideal heart rate is 60–75 per cent of that number. Now we know that many people can sustain aerobic exercise at higher heart rates. Perhaps the best way to know whether you're meeting your exercise goal is to rank the activity like this:

- ✔ Very, very light
- ✔ Very light
- ✔ Fairly light
- ✔ Somewhat hard
- ✔ Very hard
- ✔ Very, very hard

If you stay at the level of 'somewhat hard' while you get into shape, you are doing the right amount of aerobic exercise.

Aim to sustain aerobic exercise for 20 to 30 minutes every day. Despite the normal loss of exercise capacity with ageing, doing this amount helps you maximise what you have and may add significant time to your life.

Don't forget to do muscle strengthening exercises as well. Using light weights of 10–15 pounds, three times a week, try three or four different exercises to work your arms and legs and strengthen your back.

Introducing Leptin: The New Hormone on the Block

Leptin, which was first described in 1994, has an important role in normal thyroid function. A hormone made in fat cells, leptin plays a major role in regulating body weight. As your body fat goes up, the leptin in your body increases, as it's made in fat cells.

When fasting, a person has a fall in T3 and TSH. This fall may result from a reduction in leptin levels as fat stores decline over time. In the future, the use of leptin may help to promote increased weight loss in obese individuals.

This section explains the brief history of our knowledge of leptin and what we know so far about its relationship with thyroid hormone.

Understanding the functions of leptin

A certain strain of obese rats has a genetic mutation that means they can't make leptin. When these rats are given leptin, they reduce their food intake, lose weight, and bounce around with increased energy levels. The same thing happens when leptin is given to normal-weight mice – they lose fat mass. Not surprisingly, scientists then looked for leptin in human beings and discovered it, hailing the gene that codes for it in our DNA as the obesity gene. Unfortunately, giving humans injections of leptin doesn't lead to substantial weight loss.

Human obesity is not usually the result of a genetic mutation in the leptin gene. However, several families do have a mutation of the leptin gene that leads to severe obesity at a young age. This gene is a recessive trait, meaning that family members with only one abnormal leptin gene instead of two do not show the disease. When people with the disease are given leptin, they experience significant weight loss and the reversal of metabolic abnormalities.

Further studies show that leptin is doing more than just signalling the body that it has too much fat. When researchers compare body-fat percentages and leptin levels in women and men, women are found to have leptin levels that are as much as two to three times higher than in men. But even though women typically have more fat mass than men, this factor does not fully explain the difference. Scientists now know that the female sex hormone, oestrogen, stimulates leptin production, while the male sex hormone, testosterone, suppresses leptin.

Researchers also know that girls go into puberty when they reach a certain weight. Puberty begins when a hormone from the hypothalamus, a part of the brain, is made for the first time. This hormone is called *gonadotrophin-releasing hormone (GnRH)*. What signals the release of GnRH? You've guessed it – leptin is now known to trigger puberty as it provides a sure sign that the fat mass is sufficient for puberty to begin.

Interacting with thyroid hormone

Leptin also interacts with several other hormones in the body, especially insulin, which appears to have an important place in regulating leptin secretion. Leptin interacts with the adrenal glands and growth hormone as well. Because thyroid hormone increases the metabolic rate and increases body temperature, researchers thought that leptin (which also regulates metabolism and body temperature) might interact with thyroid hormone.

Leptin is now known to help regulate the part of the brain that releases thyrotrophin-releasing hormone (TRH), and to regulate the release of thyroid-stimulating hormone (TSH). When a person fasts, both their thyroid hormone and leptin concentrations fall. If leptin is given to the fasting individual, their TSH and the T4 hormone return to normal.

On the other hand, thyroid hormone also controls leptin production to some extent. In animals without thyroids, leptin concentration is increased, but when thyroid hormone is replaced, leptin levels are suppressed. Understanding of the role of leptin is at an early stage and its full role in thyroid disease is still not clear; stay tuned.

Chapter 16

Helping Yourself: Herbs and Homeopathy

• •

In This Chapter

▶ Using complementary medicine

▶ Finding a therapist

▶ Treating thyroid problems with herbs

▶ Combating thyroid problems with homeopathic remedies

• •

Complementary medicine is now mainstream, and most supermarkets and pharmacies sell homeopathic and herbal remedies, not just health food shops. Many orthodox doctors now suggest complementary remedies to their patients, such as glucosamine sulphate for arthritis and St John's wort for depression. Few suggest remedies to help thyroid problems, however. This reason is primarily because research has not yet looked into their effectiveness. But lack of evidence of effectiveness is not the same as evidence of lack of efficacy. Mostly, the research is unavailable because it's not worth anyone's while to fund it. As a result, many remedies traditionally used to treat thyroid problems are based on years of anecdotal evidence of their benefit, rather than scientific studies. The use of some remedies is also based on common sense, in that they are good sources of iodine, or have a calming action.

Although herbal remedies are not yet available on the National Health Service (NHS), you can obtain an NHS prescription for homeopathic remedies, assuming that you consult an NHS general practitioner (GP) who is trained in this method. The NHS also funds five homeopathic hospitals in the United Kingdom.

Finding a Reputable Practitioner

A variety of healers practise herbal medicine and/or homeopathy including homeopaths, naturopaths, chiropractors, osteopaths, herbalists, dentists, acupuncturists, and even GPs. Experience and training vary widely, however, and selecting a therapist who carries professional indemnity insurance is important. To find an accredited medical herbalist, contact the National Institute of Medical Herbalists at www.nimh.org.uk. You can also search www.irch.org, the International Register of Consultant Herbalists and Homeopaths.

You are entitled to homeopathic treatment on the NHS, and if your doctor decides that it's appropriate, he can refer you to an NHS doctor at one of the five NHS homeopathic hospitals, or at an NHS homeopathic clinic. If your doctor refuses to refer you, ask him to discuss their reasons and to explain why they do not feel the treatment is appropriate. You can then request a second opinion. The British Homeopathic Association publish a useful guide called 'How to get Homeopathic Treatment on the NHS', which you can request by phone on 0870 444 3950, Email: info@trusthomeopathy.org or by visiting www.trusthomeopathy.org, the Association's Web site.

Homeopathic remedies prescribed by a medically trained homeopathic doctor on a normal NHS prescription form are dispensed at homeopathic pharmacies for the usual prescription charge or exemptions. You can also consult a private homeopathic practitioner. To find an accredited homeopath visit www.trusthomeopathy.org, the Web site of the Faculty of Homeopathy.

You can also search www.irch.org, the Web site ofthe International Register of Consultant Herbalists and Homeopaths.

If you decide to consult a complementary practitioner, ask them the following questions before committing yourself to an appointment:

- Where did you study?
- What are your qualifications?
- What is your experience in treating thyroid problems?
- What does treatment consist of?
- What benefits can I expect from your treatment?
- How long does your treatment last?
- How much does it cost?

If you decide to consult a complementary therapist, do keep your doctor informed about any treatments you're taking. It's also a good idea to check with a pharmacist for any interactions between the conventional drugs you are taking and any herbal remedies your therapist suggests you start taking.

Digging into Medicinal Herbs

Herbal medicine uses different parts of different plants – leaves, roots, bark, sap, fruit, seeds, or flowers – for medicinal purposes. Herbs are either eaten in their natural form, or dried and ground to produce a powder that's made into a watery infusion (tea or *tisane*), an alcoholic solution (*tincture*), or packed as raw powder into tablets/capsules. Increasingly, active ingredients are extracted using a solvent, which is then removed to produce a more concentrated extract used to make tablets or capsules.

Solid extracts are described according to their concentration so that, for example, a 10:1 extract means ten parts (for example 10 grams) of raw herb was used to make one part (in this example 1 gram) of final extract. Although it seems logical that more concentrated herbal extracts have a more powerful action, this is not always the case. Sometimes, active ingredients evaporate away, so in fact the final concentrate is actually weaker. Because of this, you find selecting a standardised preparation, where possible, is better. Standardisation means that each batch provides a standardised or consistent amount of selected active ingredients, and brings the same benefit.

Herbs used to treat thyroid problems generally fall into one of four main groups and either:

✔ Help to normalise body functions, and help you adapt to different situations (and are known as *adaptogens*)

✔ Are good sources of iodine

✔ Have a calming action

✔ Or, have an anti-inflammatory action

Medical herbalists often use one or more of the following herbs to treat thyroid problems. They are best used under medical supervision only.

Bladderwrack

Despite its name, bladderwrack (*Fucus vesiculosus*) is not for those with problems with their waterworks. Bladderwrack is a form of kelp seaweed that is named after its bulbous floatation devices. A rich source of iodine, bladderwrack is suggested for people with an underactive thyroid that is linked with lack of iodine. Short-term studies show that taking kelp as a dietary supplement increases levels of TSH.

Bugleweed

Bugleweed (*Lycopus virginicus*) and its closer relative Gipsywort (*Lycopus europaeus*) are traditionally used to treat mild forms of hyperthyroidism. Some research suggests they can reduce production of TSH and lower thyroid hormone levels. They are also used to improve heart function.

Do not take Bugleweed or Gipsywort if you have an underactive thyroid, or if you have thyroid enlargement without changes in thyroid function. Do not take with other thyroid medication. Suddenly stopping these herbs can lead to increased production of TSH and an increase in hyperthyroid symptoms. These conditions are all good reasons why these (and other herbs) are only used under professional supervision in people with thyroid problems.

Korean ginseng

Korean ginseng (*Panax ginseng*) roots are one of the oldest known herbal medicines, used in the Orient as a revitalising and life-enhancing tonic for over 7,000 years. Ginseng roots contain at least 28 different ginsenosides, some of which are calming and relaxing, while others are more stimulating. Ginseng helps the body adapt to physical or emotional stress and has a normalising effect on hormone imbalances. Korean ginseng is used to help treat an underactive thyroid gland. Chinese studies suggest that taking ginseng extracts for two weeks can significantly increase T3 and T4 levels. You traditionally take this herb cyclically – for example, in a two weeks on, two weeks off cycle.

Motherwort

Motherwort (*Leonurus cardiaca*) is taken for many different conditions. This herb is used to regulate the heartbeat, and to reduce palpitations and levels of thyroid hormone in people with an overactive thyroid gland. However, people with thyroid problems need careful assessment before using this herb, as it may interfere with orthodox treatment.

Oats

Oatstraw (*Avena sativa*) is a popular, restorative nerve tonic. It's used to help treat nervous exhaustion and stress. It helps to boost stamina in people with an underactive thyroid gland, while calming those with an overactive thyroid.

Siberian ginseng

Siberian ginseng (*Eleutherococcus senticosus*) has similar properties to Korean ginseng. It's often regarded as an inexpensive substitute for Korean ginseng, but many researchers consider this herb a more remarkable *adaptogen* (helps to normalise body functions) with a higher activity and wider range of therapeutic uses. Siberian ginseng is traditionally used to normalise and support thyroid function whether the gland is overactive or underactive.

Turmeric

Turmeric (*Curcuma longa*) is the orange spice that makes curry mixtures so yellow. It contains an anti-inflammatory substance called *curcumin* that has an action similar to that of the steroid drug, hydrocortisone. Research suggests that turmeric helps to stimulate thyroid function and can increase production of T3 and T4 – even when given together with an antithyroid drug. Turmeric is used to support thyroid function, especially in people with an underactive gland linked with an autoimmune problem.

Valerian

People with an overactive thyroid gland often have symptoms of anxiety and can experience sleep problems such as insomnia (see chapter 2). Valerian (*Valeriana officinalis*) is one of the most calming herbs available. It calms nervous anxiety and promotes sleep. Valerian contains a number of unique substances (for example, valeric acid) that are thought to raise levels of an inhibitory brain chemical, gamma-aminobutyric acid (GABA), to damp down over-anxiety. Among 125 people in one trial, those taking valerian extracts fell asleep more quickly and woke up less often during the night than those taking a placebo. Another study shows that valerian extracts produce beneficial effects on sleep quality and duration.

If you wish to take a herbal remedy and have a thyroid problem, always consult a medical herbalist. He can advise which herbs are likely to suit you best, at which dose, without interfering with any medication you're taking. Importantly, tell your doctor if you take herbal remedies.

Understanding Homeopathy

Unlike herbal remedies that contain a known quantity of active ingredients, homeopathic remedies do not contain any measurable active ingredients. They are made according to the homeopathic principles that 'like cures like' and 'less cures more'.

The idea behind homeopathy was developed by Dr Samuel Hahnemann in the 18th century. He reasoned that, if large amounts of a substance can cause symptoms of a disease in a healthy person, then very small amounts of the same substance can help the body get better, rather like a vaccine. Tiny amounts of a substance are selected that, if given neat, produce similar symptoms to those they are designed to treat. Instead, they are diluted many hundreds of thousands of times to leave a medicinal 'footprint' that prompts the body to heal itself.

Not only does a homeopath find out about your symptoms, he also wants to know about your personality, likes and dislikes, emotions, family history, and what makes your symptoms better, or worse. This information helps to pinpoint your constitutional type – which has a bearing on which remedies suit you best.

Discovering homeopathic remedies

Homeopathic remedies are derived from a variety of sources: leaves, berries, fruits, bark, roots, minerals, and sometimes animals – even snakes and spiders!

In keeping with the idea that small amounts are best, remedies are diluted over and over again. And each time they're diluted, they are shaken and struck in a special way known as *succussion*. The more they are diluted, shaken, and struck, the stronger they are. In fact, a homoeopathic remedy may only contain one part per million of the active ingredient that is believed to leave behind a molecular memory within the water molecules used for dilution, in a similar way that a musical memory is recorded in iron molecules on a magnetic tape.

Remedies are rated according to their potency. When one drop of the medicinal substance is shaken and struck into 99 drops of *diluent* (the liquid in which it is being dissolved), the remedy has a potency rating of 1c. If one drop is taken out of this mixture and added to 99 drops of new diluent, the new remedy has a potency rating of 2c. If one drop of the 2c remedy is then diluted with 99 drops of a new diluent, the potency rating rises to 3c, and so on.

- **Low potency remedies:** Up to 6c, are used when only physical symptoms or severe changes in the disease state exist.

- **Medium potency remedies:** From 12c to 30c, are used when physical and mental or emotional symptoms exist.

- **High potency remedies:** Up to 200c or greater, are used when the problem is long-standing or severe.

Taking a remedy

When you have a thyroid problem, see a trained homeopath who can assess your constitutional type as well as your symptoms before deciding which treatment is right for you.

Homeopathic medicines are ideally taken on their own, without eating or drinking for at least 30 minutes before or afterwards. Tablets are also taken without handling – tip them into the lid of the container, or onto a teaspoon to transfer them to your mouth. Then suck or chew them, don't swallow them whole.

When taking homeopathic remedies, avoid drinking strong tea or coffee if possible as these may interfere with the homeopathic effect.

Occasionally, symptoms initially get worse before they get better. This stage is known as *aggravation*. Although aggravation is uncommon, try to persevere as it's a good sign that the remedy is working. After completing a course of homoeopathy, you usually feel better in yourself with a greatly improved sense of wellbeing that lets you cope with any remaining symptoms in a more positive way.

The following remedies are often suggested for people with thyroid problems, and are taken together with any prescribed drugs they need.

Arsenicum album

Made from the white, poisonous metallic salt, arsenic oxide, this remedy is useful for anxiety, diarrhoea, and burning heat. It's especially helpful for people whose constitutional type is associated with thinness, worry lines, restlessness, and with quick movements. These symptoms and signs are similar to those that can occur with hyperthyroidism, in fact. Sometimes, the remedy is also suggested for people with an underactive thyroid gland.

Iodum

As its name suggests, iodum is made from iodine. Iodum is mainly used to treat symptoms associated with an overactive thyroid gland, including eye pain, enlarged goitre, and a ravenous appetite together with a tendency to lose weight and sweat a lot.

Belladonna

Belladonna is made from the herb, deadly nightshade (*Atropa belladonna*). It's used to treat complaints with a sudden onset, including fever, staring eyes, and a red, hot, flushed face. This property makes Belladonna suitable for some people with an overactive thyroid gland.

Natrum Mur

Natrum muriaticum is made from sodium chloride – common table salt. It has a wide range of uses, including constipation, general feelings of illness, chilliness, and slowing down. This remedy is useful for people with an underactive thyroid gland, especially if their constitutional type is associated with paleness, puffiness, seriousness, and slow movements.

If you find a herbal or homeopathic remedy helpful, let your doctor know. This feedback may encourage your doctor to suggest a natural approach to another patient who continues to have problems while using orthodox medicine alone.

Part IV
Special Considerations in Thyroid Health

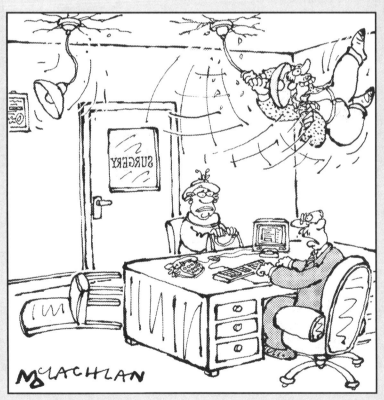

"We think your husband's overactive state is due to hyperthyroidism."

In this part . . .

Certain groups are affected differently from the rest of us by thyroid disease. These include pregnant women, children, and elderly people. Their special needs are taken up in this part.

Also, we talk you through the genetic link to thyroid diseases and what scientists are doing to try to prevent their transmission from one generation to the next.

Chapter 17

Examining the Genetic Link to Thyroid Disease

Chapters 2, 5, and 6 introduce you to several members of one family: Sarah, Margaret, Stacy, Karen, and Tammy. The reason these five women all come from the same prestigious family is that thyroid diseases are often hereditary. Many (though not all) thyroid diseases have a genetic link.

This chapter discusses the various thyroid diseases you can inherit and how they pass from one generation to the next. Progress in understanding the inheritance of thyroid disease is nothing short of amazing, but all this new information makes the subject pretty complicated.

In all honesty, this subject isn't for the faint-hearted. If you're interested in knowing how your genes promote the development of certain diseases, this chapter is perfect for tickling your intellect. If you're reading this book solely to determine how to treat your present thyroid condition, you may want to skip this chapter entirely. But, even if the term genetics strikes fear in your heart, you may find the end of the chapter (the section called 'The Future of Managing Hereditary Thyroid Disease') interesting as it tells you about the exciting ways in which scientists are attempting to prevent thyroid disease and many other conditions with a genetic basis.

Genetics for Beginners

To understand how genetic disease affects the thyroid, you need a basic understanding of genetics. This section provides all the background you need, though as it's not a book about genetics, this section is as brief as possible while still giving you the essentials.

A monk and his pea plants

Although he didn't achieve celebrity status during his lifetime, Gregor Mendel, an Austrian monk, is the starting point for all the great discoveries in genetics, the science of heredity. Mendel studied pea plants, looking at how various characteristics of these plants are passed on, such as height, seed texture (smooth or wrinkled), pod shape (plump or pinched) and so on.

Mendel knew that pea plants form new seeds when pollen in the male part of the plant (the anther) manages to attach to the female part (the stigma) and get down to the ovaries, which house the eggs which it fertilizes. The result is a seed, which grows into a plant.

Mendel carefully controlled the fertilization of his pea plants so he knew exactly which plant provided the pollen and which plant provided the ovary. He took, for example, the pollen of short pea plants that never produce anything but short pea plants, and used it to fertilize the ovaries of tall pea plants that never produce anything but tall pea plants. Then he took the pollen from tall pea plants and fertilized the ovaries of short pea plants. The result, in both cases, was always tall pea plants.

Mendel then took the tall offspring from this first fertilization (called the first cross) and fertilised them with each other. The offspring of the second cross were not all tall: Three-fourths were tall, and one-fourth was short. When Mendel crossed (or ferilised) the short plants from the second cross with other short plants from the second cross, the resulting plants were always short. But if he crossed the short ones with the tall plants from the second cross, the new plants were usually, but not always, tall. The same pattern held true for the other characteristics that Mendel studied.

On the basis of these studies, Mendel made the following observations in the pea plant:

- A feature of the pollen and the egg determines whether a plant is tall or short. (This feature is now called a gene; Mendel did not use this term.)

- When the gene from the tall plant combines with the gene from the short plant, they do not mix to form an average plant.

- If a plant has two characteristics for the same gene such as tallness and shortness, one is found more often than the other when they are crossed. (The gene that produces the trait found more often is the *dominant* gene, and the gene producing the trait found less often is the *recessive* gene.)

✔ There are two different genes for a trait. (Two genes that determine the same trait are called *alleles.*)

✔ When plants with two different traits such as height and texture of the seed are bred, these traits pass to the offspring independently of one another. For example, a tall plant isn't always found with a smooth seed or always with a wrinkled seed. Mendel concluded that genes (which he called *atoms of inheritance*) follow the principle of *independent assortment:* Each trait is inherited separately from all other traits.

Mendel's work received little attention when it announced in 1865, but luckily, it was rediscovered in 1900, and he got posthumous credit for his discoveries (for what that was worth).

Talk the talk

Using Mendel's research as a basis, scientists created the new language of genetics which makes it difficult to understand what they are talking about.

First, if a person (or a plant, dog, or chimpanzee) has two copies of the same allele, he or she is *homozygous* for that gene. If he or she has one of each allele, the person is *heterozygous* for that gene. (We now know that, within a population, there are more than two different alleles for each gene. However, any given person, animal, or plant has only two alleles for each gene.)

The appearance of the trait due to particular genes is called the *phenotype,* while the genes that make up that phenotype are called the *genotype.* For instance, two tall pea plants with the same appearance (phenotype) can have a different genotype. A plant with only tall genes is tall, but so is a plant with a tall gene and a short gene (because tallness is the dominant gene).

A quick quiz: Based on your in-depth knowledge of genetics, can two short pea plants have different genotypes? The answer is no, because shortness is the recessive gene. If a tallness gene is thrown into the mix, the plant is tall. Therefore, all short pea plants can only have the genes for shortness.

The great divide

While the world was ignoring Mendel's work, great things were happening under the microscope. Scientists saw that tissues are made up of cells and that new cells come from the division of old cells. As two new cells form, the old cell produces two copies of everything so that each new cell contains exactly what the old cell had.

One particular area of the cell, which looks like a cell within the cell, is especially intriguing to scientists. This area is called the *nucleus* of the cell. As two new cells are formed, some substances in the nucleus double and separate so that each new cell gets a complete set of these substances, which are called *chromosomes*.

Scientists now know that each plant and animal has a set of chromosomes, but the numbers of chromosomes often differs between species. For instance, humans have 23 pairs or 46 chromosomes, while chimpanzees have 24 pairs or 48 chromosomes. (But chimpanzee chromosomes look more like human chromosomes than ape chromosomes, so don't start thinking you're so smart.) The whole process in which one cell becomes two is called *mitosis*.

Through examining the division of egg cells and sperm cells (the so-called *germ cells*), scientists know that each of these cells contains only half the normal number of chromosomes. In humans, for example, each egg cell and each sperm cell has one set of 23 chromosomes (while other human cells have 46 chromosomes). When these cells divide to form more sperm or egg cells (through a process called meiosis), the result is again 23 chromosomes per cell. When the egg and the sperm join together in fertilization, the combination, called a *zygote*, has the normal number of 46 chromosomes.

When a zygote is formed, one set of its chromosomes comes from the female (mother) and one set of chromosomes comes from the male (father). In the zygote cell, these chromosomes pair up two-by-two. The members of each chromosome pair are called *homologous chromosomes*.

As is always the case, there's an exception to this rule. But like the French say, 'vive le difference'. Very loosely translated, that means 'Thank goodness for this particular set of chromosomes.' This unique set is the sex chromosomes that determine whether you are a boy or a girl. All other pairs of chromosomes have matched genes so that if there's a gene for a given characteristic on one of the chromosomes of the pair, the other chromosome also has a gene for that characteristic. While a female has two matched sex chromosomes (called X chromosomes), a male has two different sex chromosomes (called an X chromosome and a Y chromosome).

Genes, chromosomes, and the traits they create

You are probably thinking, 'Two genes for every trait, two sets of chromosomes . . . genes and chromosomes are the same.' The problem is that any given plant, animal, or human has far more traits than the number of chromosomes they own. Recognizing this, scientists realized that each chromosome contains many genes, not just one.

Each gene for a particular trait is found on a single chromosome. Each chromosome is passed down to its daughter cells – the cells they create when that cell divides. Therefore, some genes (and the traits they create) get passed down together from generation to generation. (They don't follow the principle of independent assortment.) Geneticists described genes on the same chromosome as linked.

Even though some genes are linked, they sometimes do get inherited independently, just as Mendel predicted. This happens because *crossing over* takes place. What is crossing over? During the process of meiosis, which produces sperm and egg cells, as the sets of chromosomes line up close together, genes on one chromosome can cross over to the other while the alleles they replace cross over in the other direction. In this way, *recombinant chromosomes* form – new combinations that help to make your offspring different from you.

The discovery of crossing over means that scientists can now map chromosomes. That is, they can determine which genes are on which chromosomes and where, because the closer two genes are, the less likely they are separated by a cross-over, while the farther they are from one another, the more likely they are to separate.

Another way that a new trait replaces an old one is when a *mutation* takes place. As a result of faulty copying of the chromosome or an outside influence such as radiation, chemicals, or the sun, a slightly different code appears in the genetic material, so that a new gene replaces an old one. A gene provides all the information needed for a cell to make a particular protein. If the code changes due to a mutation, this means a different amino acid sequence is inserted into that protein. Usually mutation isn't noticed, either because the different amino acid sequence doesn't affect the function of the protein, or because the mutation kills the individual so that it isn't reproduced. Once in a while, a mutation is good for the animal or plant in which it occurs, producing a useful trait such as blue-coloured roses instead of white.

The secret lives of genes

Genes are made up of long, long, long chains of nucleic acids. Nucleic acids have three components: a sugar called deoxyribose; a phosphate attached at one end of the sugar; and a base (one of adenine, cytosine, guanine, or thymine) attached to the sugar at another point. The long chemical structure from which genes are made is known as deoxyribonucleic acid or DNA.

DNA

Within the DNA, the number of adenine molecules is always equal to the number of thymine molecules, while the cytosine equals the guanine. In 1952, biochemists James Watson and Francis Crick showed that this equality is because each gene contains two chains of nucleic acids. The adenine on one chain is always paired with the thymine on the other, while cytosine on one chain is always paired with guanine on the other. As DNA has a helical structure, Watson and Crick called the structure a double helix – a shape that looks like a spiral staircase.

One of the best things about the identification of the double helix is that it became clear how genes copy themselves or replicate. The helix simply breaks apart into two strands. Each of the two strands then act as a template so that a new strand forms on it in the only way it can, so that a nucleic acid containing adenine connects to a nucleic acid containing thymine, and a nucleic acid containing cytosine connects with a nucleic acid containing guanine. The result is two new double helixes.

Next, DNA acts as a blueprint to control the creation of the animal or plant and the ongoing processes that allow it to live. This function is carried out using ribonucleic acid, or RNA.

RNA

RNA is made up of nucleic acids just like DNA, but the sugar in RNA is ribose and the bases are adenine, cytosine, and guanine, with uracil replacing thymine.

RNA forms against the DNA template in the same way that the double helix breaks apart to reproduce itself. When a gene is active, the DNA containing that gene splits apart and a strand of RNA is made with the gene providing the template. This copying process is called transcription. The RNA molecule is essentially a copy of the gene but made up of RNA instead of DNA. The RNA remains as a single strand, not a double helix, and is called messenger RNA (mRNA) because it carries the message from the DNA to the next level of control, the *ribosome*. Ribosomes are small dumb-bell-shaped factories found in each cell which take in the strip of RNA instructions and read it, rather like ticker-tape, churning out a protein at the other end. This process is called translation.

Proteins

Proteins are made up of amino acids. Every three bases in the messenger RNA, called a *triplet*, causes one particular amino acid to line up opposite them within the ribosome. Each group of three bases is called a *codon*, and each codon codes for a specific amino acid. Scientists use artificial messenger RNA containing the same codon again and again to determine which amino acid is selected by each codon.

With four different bases, each of which can occur at any of the three sites in a codon, the maximum number of codon combinations that are possible is $4 \times 4 \times 4 = 64$. But, there are only 20 amino acids, not 64. Researchers now know that several different codons select the same amino acid, and that some codons act as the code for the end of a protein, without selecting an amino acid. They form the genetic equivalent of a full stop at the end of a messenger RNA sentence.

 Just to complicate things a little further, amino acids don't actually line up opposite the codons but are carried at one end of another RNA molecule called transfer RNA. At its other end, transfer RNA has the bases that are complementary to the codon. So the transfer RNA lines up neatly against the messenger RNA, within the ribosome, while the amino acids are lined up next to one another at the other end. A series of other steps then bind the amino acids into a protein.

Shall I form a liver or a brain?

As we mentioned (see 'The great divide' earlier in this chapter) a fertilized egg reproduces itself in a process called mitosis, which creates two identical cells. These cells divide and divide again until a complex human being develops. So how do these identical cells transform themselves into a thyroid cell, a liver cell or even a brain cell which are very different from each other?

Even though each cell contains an identical set of genes, not all these genes are active. In some cells, certain genes are switched on, so that certain proteins are made, while other genes are switched off. A thyroid cell differs from a brain cell as a result of the particular genes that are *expressed* (active) in each cell. Many different factors determine whether a gene is expressed or not, such as the presence of various hormones or growth factors that are allowed to enter some cells but not others.

The expression of a gene is sometimes controlled at the level of the gene itself, while at other times the gene happily transcribes itself to make messenger RNA, but for some reason the cell ignores that type of mRNA and the protein it codes for is never made. In these and in many other ways still undiscovered, cells use only the genes they need to function within their environment.

The Origins of Genetic Thyroid Diseases

This understanding of genetics helps to explain how some thyroid diseases are transmitted through inheritance. A child inherits a thyroid disease in one of three ways:

✔ A single gene from a parent may transmit a dominant or recessive trait to the child. This is the method Mendel recognised with his peas.

✔ Often, many genes are involved in the inheritance of a disease so the child has to inherit all of them to get the disease.

✔ An abnormality affecting an entire chromosome may result in disease. For example, if a female ends up with only one X chromosome, instead of two, that lack produces a condition known as Turner's syndrome, which often includes a thyroid disorder.

Inheriting a disease through a single gene

Many diseases are inherited through a single gene, often as a result of a gene mutation. If the disease is inherited as a recessive gene, both parents must supply the same gene in order for the disease to appear. If it is inherited as a dominant gene, only one parent supplies the gene necessary to cause the disease. Alternatively, if a disease is inherited with the X chromosome in a recessive form, then only a male can get the disease, as he has just one X chromosome (paired with a Y chromosome), while a female is spared unless both her X chromosomes carry the gene.

The entire list of diseases transmitted by single-gene inheritance may be found at `http://www.ncbi.nlm.nih.gov/entrez/query.fcgi?db=OMIM`, the homepage of Online Mendelian Inheritance in Man (OMIM), a huge database compiled by Dr. Victor McKusick at Johns Hopkins University. If you search the term 'thyroid' from the homepage, 559 different thyroid diseases are listed at the time of writing. Each one is fully described, with citations for all the research that has helped to define the defect and a complete bibliography at the end of each description.

Recessive inheritance

Many conditions in which thyroid hormone isn't made properly fall into the category of recessive inheritance. It takes two 'bad' genes to develop one of these conditions. If you have just one bad gene, you're a carrier of the disease, but you don't experience it yourself. The phenotype (the way this genetic pattern makes itself known) is usually a large thyroid that doesn't produce sufficient thyroid hormone. Although several conditions appear similar, in that the final result is absence of thyroid hormone, each condition involves a defect at a different step in thyroid hormone production. Among the conditions inherited this way are:

✔ *A defect in the production of thyroid hormone* (see Chapter 3): People with this condition are hypothyroid (see Chapter 5) and have goitres. This condition stems from an abnormality in the creation of the enzyme that produces thyroid hormone.

✔ *Thyroid hormone unresponsiveness:* If you inherit a bad gene instead of the gene that makes the receptor protein for thyroid hormone, your cells are not responsive to the thyroid hormone your body produces. People with this condition are deaf and have goitres. With this condition, the T3, T4, and TSH levels are all elevated (see Chapter 4).

✔ *Pendred Syndrome:* People with this disease are deaf and have goitres, but their thyroid function is normal. The disease also causes mental impairment and an increased tendency to develop thyroid cancer. The defect is in the production of thyroid hormone, but at some point it improves so that hypothyroidism isn't present later on.

✔ *Thyroid transcription factor defect:* People affected have a goitre and decreased levels of thyroglobulin. *Transcription* is the term for the production of messenger RNA from DNA, which is where this defect arises.

✔ *Defect in thyroid production:* This is different from *thyroid* transcription factor defect. Someone with this condition is hypothyroid, has a goitre, and experiences mental impairment. Lab tests show a defect in the formation of thyroid hormone. Normally, two molecules of tyrosine with iodine attached couple together to form thyroid hormone, but this process fails in this particular inherited condition.

Dominant inheritance

Many inherited thyroid conditions are passed from parents to children this way: Only one 'bad' gene is needed to produce this disease. These diseases are more common than those inherited by recessive genes, and examples include:

✔ *A thyroid hormone receptor defect:* If you have this condition, your body is resistant to the action of thyroid hormones. At the same time, you experience mild hyperthyroidism. People with this condition have short stature, learning disabilities, deafness, and a goitre. Lab tests show high levels of T3, T4, and TSH.

✔ *Papillary thyroid carcinoma* (see Chapter 8): This type of cancer usually occurs at an earlier age than thyroid cancer that isn't inherited.

✔ *A different defect in thyroid hormone receptor:* This produces a child with severe cretinism of the neurologic form (see Chapter 12).

✔ *Thyroid hormone resistance* (also found in a recessive form): Someone with this condition has a goitre and as a child begins to speak at a later than expected age, but thyroid function is normal. Lab tests show that T3 and T4 levels are high, but the TSH level is normal.

✔ *Multiple Endocrine Neoplasia, Type II:* This condition causes tumours in multiple organs, including medullary carcinoma of the thyroid (see Chapter 8), a tumour of the adrenal glands, and tumours of the parathyroid glands. Lab tests show increased levels of epinephrine (adrenaline) and calcitonin in the blood.

✔ *Medullary Carcinoma of the Thyroid, Familial:* People with this condition have medullary cancer (see Chapter 8).

X-linked inheritance

X-linked inheritance presents fewer examples because men have only one X chromosome and women have two, compared to 44 other chromosomes that can produce a disease by recessive or dominant inheritance. If a disease passed on with the X chromosome is recessive, both parents must give the gene to a daughter in order for the disease to appear, but a son gets the disease if only one parent passes along the gene (as he only has one X chromosome, paired against a Y). These conditions are therefore much more common in males. Some examples of diseases inherited this way include:

✔ *Immunodeficiency and Polyendocrinopathy:* A baby with this condition has unmanageable diarrhoea, diabetes, and thyroid autoimmune disease. Sadly, a child born with this condition often dies very young.

✔ *Thyroid-binding globulin abnormality:* This condition produces mental disability. Lab tests show that someone with this disease has decreased thyroid-binding globulin (see Chapter 3).

✔ *Multinodular goitre:* The thyroid is larger and multinodular (see Chapter 9).

Inherited thyroid diseases can affect every step in thyroid hormone production, transportation, and action. The ones listed here are only 14 of the 559 currently listed in the OMIM database, and new conditions are discovered all the time.

Inheriting a disease through multiple genes

Autoimmune thyroiditis is the major thyroid disease that is inherited as a result of abnormalities of multiple genes. This disease is much more common in women than men, so it seems likely that the inheritance is linked to the

X chromosome. If this is the case, the method in which the X chromosome passes the disease along isn't yet known. Another idea is that the female sex hormone, oestrogen, influences the occurrence of this disease, but just how this may happen isn't understood.

Autoimmune thyroiditis is easy to diagnose because lab tests show that a person has autoantibodies (see Chapter 5) that damage the thyroid. Many genes are involved in the production of autoantibodies. The substance (such as thyroid tissue) that provokes antibodies is called an antigen. The antigen is first broken into small pieces that are bound to special proteins on cell membranes called major histocompatibility molecules. These molecules are involved in recognising self antigens from non-self antigens, so the immune system doesn't normally attack the body's own components. When a non-self antigen combines with these proteins, it leads to the activation of another cell called the T cell. The T cell helps yet another cell, the B cell, recognize the foreign antigens and produce antibodies against it. Multiple genes are involved in all these steps.

The major histocompatibility region of the chromosomes is on the short arm of chromosome 6. It determines which self antigens are found on white blood cells. These self antigens are the human leukocyte antigens (HLA). Using chemicals to identify these self antigens, scientists have found that in Caucasians, HLA-B8 and HLA-DR3 are the antigens most associated with Graves' disease (see Chapter 6), while in Koreans, the DR5 and DR8 are most common. In Japanese, the antigen most associated with Graves' disease is DR5, and in Chinese, it's DR9. All of this is important because doctors can test for these antigens in relatives of affected individuals. If the antigens are present, they are more likely to get the disease.

Another disease that is found more often in people with certain human leukocyte antigens is postpartum thyroiditis (see Chapter 11). In Caucasians, the antigens involved are HLA DR3, DR4, or DR5, while in Chinese, it is DR9.

Inheriting a chromosome abnormality

As new cells are formed during the creation of a zygote (fertilised egg), it's possible for a mistake to occur when chromosomes are divided between two new cells so that one cell ends up with an extra chromosome and the other ends up with one less chromosome. The most well-known conditions associated with this kind of chromosome mistake are Turner's syndrome and Down's syndrome. Down's syndrome results when new cells contain three copies of the 21st chromosome instead of two, while Turner's syndrome results when an X chromosome is left behind, so that cells contain one female sex chromosome instead of two. Both conditions are associated with hypothyroidism, but Down's syndrome is also associated with hyperthyroidism on occasion.

The Future of Managing Hereditary Thyroid Disease

Up until now, scientists have not had much success in their attempts to remove a 'bad' gene from a human and replace it with a healthy gene – a process known as genetic engineering. The main problem is in delivering the new gene successfully. As soon as scientists determine how to do this, the door is open to an exciting future world in which diseases that are inherited through a single gene are readily prevented.

Genetic engineering

If a disease is due to a recessive gene, replacing that gene with its dominant form in sufficient amounts should cure the condition. Usually in a recessive gene disorder, the disease occurs because that particular gene isn't functioning at all, so providing even a small level of function may cure the condition.

Blood system disorders are expected to most easily respond to genetic engineering as blood is easily removed and replaced with a new gene spliced into the cells. The first trial of gene therapy, performed in 1990, was for a disorder that resulted in severe loss of immunity so the patient was susceptible to infections, as well as a cancer. Scientists tried connecting the necessary gene to a virus, which infected the blood cells of the patient and added the gene to their DNA. The cells were then cultured to increase their number and reinserted. Unfortunately, the trial didn't work, probably because the efficiency of splicing the gene into the cells was low.

Trials of gene therapy have also taken place for other genetic disorders, including familial hypercholesterolemia (where excessive production of cholesterol leads to heart attack); cystic fibrosis (where lack of a certain gene leads to excessive production of a thick mucus in the lungs); and Duchenne muscular dystrophy (where there is severe muscle deterioration).Unfortunately, gene replacement therapy in all three of these conditions is so far unsuccessful.

Another novel way of managing diseases caused by defective genes is to find a gene that is active during fetal life, but which becomes dormant later on. If isolated, and encouraged to express itself, such a gene might replace the activity of the defective gene. A prime candidate for this treatment is sickle cell disease in which red blood cells carry abnormal haemoglobin (the pigment that carries oxygen). As a result, they are sickle or crescent-shaped in appearance, and block blood flow to tissues, causing great pain. A gene active during fetal life produces fetal haemoglobin, which doesn't sickle. If scientists can find a way to turn on this gene during adult life, it can replace the defective haemoglobin.

Cancer treatment has seen a lot of activity in the area of gene therapy. One approach is to insert a gene that increases the sensitivity of cancer cells to a drug, or to insert a poison into cells that are then injected directly into a tumour. Another approach is to insert a gene that increases the activity of the patient's immune system. Finally, some tumours arise when the activity of tumour suppressors (chemicals in the body that suppress the growth of tumours) declines. Treatment aims to restore tumour suppressor activity with a new gene that is inserted into blood cells. All these treatments have seen some success, but no one has yet cured cancer with gene therapy. And, so far, none of the cancer therapy trials have targeted thyroid cancer.

Scientists are also attempting to increase a tumour's ability to provoke an immune response against it. To do this, scientists insert genes into the tumour that cause it to produce new antigens, which the body attacks as it recognises them as foreign. Tumours like malignant melanoma and colon cancer are the target of this type of therapy. A similar technique involves inserting a gene directly into a tumour that activates a cancer-killing agent, which is subsequently injected. These techniques have led to some decrease in tumour size but, so far, no cures. Interestingly, the use of gene therapy isn't limited to tumours that are brought on by faulty genes but are directed at any tumour, genetic or not.

The ethics of germline gene therapy

As you can see, the range of techniques for using genetic engineering to cure disease is enormous. New methods of delivering healthy genes to replace disease-conferring genes are discovered almost every day. This approach is certainly the most simple and elegant way of treating diseases provoked by inheritance of a single dominant gene. However, this type of treatment can only cure a particular individual – it doesn't affect the transmission of the disease to his or her offspring. To eliminate these diseases from future generations, genetic engineering has to take place in the sperm and/or the egg, the germline of the individual.

Germline gene therapy raises tremendous ethical questions. If we can eliminate a recessively inherited condition such as Pendred syndrome, with the replacement of a Pendred gene with a normal gene, scientists also, potentially, have the tools for changing skin colour, height, or any other body characteristic in future generations.

Although germline gene therapy is successful in some animals, it has not yet been allowed on humans for several reasons:

✔ The methods used so far are very imprecise, so the final product is uncertain, including the possible introduction of harmful genes.

✔ Many people fear that germline gene therapy may lead to germline enhancement, an attempt to produce a 'superior' human being.

✔ It's uncertain that germline gene therapy is even needed, because a harmful recessive trait requires mating with another human with the same trait to express itself, while dominant traits are present in only half of a germline. It therefore makes more sense to identify the sperm or egg with the normal gene and use that in fertilization, rather than trying to modify the sperm or egg with the abnormal gene. Genetic testing of the germline is needed to eliminate these diseases.

An entire field of genetics concerns ELSI, the ethical, legal, and social implications of genetic science.

Clearly, genetics is the current frontier in medical science. It promises to prevent or cure many of the diseases that plague humans, including hereditary thyroid disease and nonhereditary tumours, but the road to that cure is filled with cracks and bumps so expect a very uneven ride.

Chapter 18

Controlling Thyroid Disease during Pregnancy

*H*aving a thyroid disorder doesn't affect your ability to have a healthy, bouncing baby. As thyroid disease is so common among women, and as so many women have babies, thyroid disease and pregnancy often go hand in hand. Some women enter the world of pregnancy with a pre-existing thyroid condition, whether they know about it or not, while other women develop thyroid problems during, and possibly as a result of, their pregnancy.

As a developing foetus is totally dependent on its mum's thyroid hormones during early pregnancy, picking up and properly treating any thyroid problems during this stage is vital. The British Thyroid Association advice doctors to check thyroid function in pregnant women during their first antenatal booking appointment if they are at risk of a thyroid problem. This means women with:

✔ A personal history of thyroid disease

✔ Type I diabetes (which is sometimes associated with autoimmune thyroid problems)

✔ A family history of thyroid disease

✔ Symptoms that are suggestive of thyroid disease

In short, if you're pregnant and have any concerns about thyroid problems, ask your doctor for a blood test. It doesn't hurt to check. (Well, having a blood test does hurt a little, but as you're having blood taken for other routine pregnancy blood tests anyway, you won't feel any additional discomfort. Honest.)

Thinking ahead is also worth doing. If you have a known thyroid problem and are planning to try for a baby, ask your doctor to check your TSH levels first, before you conceive, so your treatment is adjusted if necessary. For example, you may need your dose of thyroxine hormone increased both before, as well as after, conceiving.

Looking at Normal Thyroid during Pregnancy

Three important changes occur in a pregnant woman's body that increase her need for iodine:

- ✔ During early pregnancy, blood flow to the kidneys is increased, resulting in lots more visits to the bathroom, and lots more iodine recycled back to the local water board.

- ✔ As the tiny foetus can't make thyroid hormones at first, the placenta – the tissue that connects the foetus to its mum – scoops up thyroid hormones from mum's circulation, so she needs to make more.

- ✔ And, even when the growing foetus does start making its own thyroid hormones, the foetus takes iodine from mum's circulation in order to do so.

At the same time, because of the extra oestrogen hormone floating around, the mother makes much more thyroxine-binding globulin – a protein that transports thyroid hormone through the blood (refer to Chapter 3) – than she used to. And, as she makes a form of thyroxine-binding globulin that leaves the circulation much more slowly than normal, she needs to make more thyroxine to make up for the increased amount that is protein bound. The bottom line is that a pregnant woman has to make more thyroid hormone than normal, so her need for iodine significantly increases.

Importantly, you need to understand all these changes if you have hypothyroidism and take thyroid hormone pills. To maintain normal thyroid function, your dose of thyroid hormone replacement usually needs to go up during early pregnancy, and the amount of adjustment needed is based on your level of thyroid-stimulating hormone (TSH). Usually, your dose of thyroxine needs to go up at least 50µg (micrograms) daily to maintain normal serum thyroid-stimulating hormone concentrations. Levels of TSH are usually assessed in every three months (trimester) of pregnancy.

While all these changes are happening, the placenta makes a lot of a special hormone called *human chorionic gonadotrophin* (HCG). This hormone maintains early pregnancy as it acts as a signal for menstrual periods to stop. Some parts of HCG are very similar to parts of TSH, and when it reaches the mother's thyroid it stimulates production of more thyroid hormone, just as TSH does. This action is rather clever of Mother Nature, as more thyroxine is exactly what is needed during early pregnancy and, as a result, the mother's level of free T4 rises, causing a fall in the amount of TSH her body produces. If she is having twins, her HCG level is especially high and can persist for weeks, causing a form of hyperthyroidism, which we discuss in the section 'Hyperthyroidism in Pregnancy' later in this chapter.

Pregnancy and Hypothyroidism

A miracle of nature takes place during pregnancy as amazingly the mother's body does not reject the foetus as a foreign intruder – which is just what happens with any other foreign invasion. (Even a few foreign cells injected inside your body wouldn't last long.)

The fact that the mother's body doesn't reject the foetus is evidence of a general decline in immunity that occurs during pregnancy. As a result, women who have autoimmune diseases prior to pregnancy often find their condition improves during pregnancy, although it usually returns to its original state again after delivery. This case is true for people with either hypothyroidism or hyperthyroidism that results from an autoimmune condition.

Decreased fertility

If a woman has untreated hypothyroidism, she can experience difficulty in conceiving as hypothyroidism decreases her fertility. In one study of infertile women in Finland, published in *Gynecological Endocrinology* in 2000, 5 per cent of women who experienced difficulty getting pregnant had previously undiagnosed hypothyroidism. In addition, if a woman with hypothyroidism does manage to achieve pregnancy, her risk of miscarriage is higher than if she didn't have a thyroid condition. And, if you are hypothyroid and are not receiving treatment with thyroid hormone replacement, your risk of obstetric complications, such as high blood pressure, problems with the placental connection to the foetus, and problems with delivery, all increase. The good news, however, is that once diagnosed and treated properly, all these risks return to normal.

Iodine deficiency

A mother with an iodine deficiency during pregnancy cannot make sufficient thyroid hormone for herself, let alone her foetus, who relies on her for thyroid hormone up until the 20th week of the pregnancy. As a result, the mother makes increasing amounts of TSH in an attempt to stimulate her thyroid, which is on a go-slow without sufficient iodine supplies. This results in the development of a goitre (refer to Chapter 9). Laboratory tests show that iodine-deficient pregnant women have:

- Reduced T4 and, if severe, reduced T3 hormone levels

- Increased TSH

- Increased ratios of T3 to T4, because the thyroid begins to prefer making T3

- Increased thyroglobulin

The mother's goitre may not fully shrink after delivery, when her iodine needs are reduced. This fact may partly explain the much greater incidence of thyroid enlargement in women compared with men.

Iodine deficiency also affects the foetus, which may develop a goitre and, sadly, may experience abnormal brain development (refer to Chapter 12).

Autoimmune hypothyroidism

In iodine-rich countries, most cases of hypothyroidism in pregnancy result from autoimmune thyroid disease.

Understanding the risks to the mother and foetus

If lab tests show that a woman has thyroid autoantibodies – even if she is not diagnosed as hypothyroid because her thyroid function tests are normal – she has a higher risk of miscarriage. Doctors are not sure why, but one suggestion is that these women really have mild hypothyroidism despite the normal test results. Another is that the autoantibodies are a sign that another autoimmune disease is present, and that this condition is what's responsible for the miscarriage.

Thyroid autoantibodies are transmitted to the foetus through the placenta, causing hypothyroidism in the foetus. Usually, if the mother is hypothyroid and is adequately treated with thyroid hormone, enough gets to the foetus to prevent this problem. If the baby is born with hypothyroidism, he or she is placed on thyroid hormone replacement until the autoantibodies are cleared from the baby's circulation, usually within three or four months. The baby does not need treatment after that.

Knowing when to treat the mother

At what point is treatment needed for autoimmune hypothyroidism in pregnancy? Usually, if a mother's TSH level is greater than 4 μU/ml (microunits per millilitre), she is treated. She then needs regular thyroid function tests throughout the pregnancy to confirm that she is receiving the right amount of thyroid medication.

If the mother's TSH level is between 2 and 4 μU/ml (microunits per millilitre), and she tests positive for thyroid autoantibodies, her doctor may decide to start treatment, and the foetus is checked for goitre or other signs of thyroid abnormality. Fortunately, recent studies show that if the mother has very mild hypothyroidism in early pregnancy, the condition has no negative effect upon the newborn's hearing or physical activity.

Although autoimmune hypothyroidism generally improves during pregnancy, the mother's hypothyroidism often worsens after the baby is born, and her T4 level may decrease further. Therefore, checking her TSH every six to eight weeks after delivery is important.

If you have hypothyroidism during pregnancy, make sure your thyroid function is checked about two months after delivery to confirm you are taking the right dose of thyroid hormone.

Certain drugs that are commonly taken during pregnancy, such as sucralfate, and aluminium hydroxide (refer to Chapter 10), can block the absorption of thyroid hormone. These drugs should be taken several hours before or after the thyroid hormone is taken.

Hyperthyroidism in Pregnancy

Two main conditions are responsible for hyperthyroidism in pregnancy: Graves' disease and a condition called gestational transient thyrotoxicosis. Regardless of the cause, the symptoms of hyperthyroidism in pregnancy include rapid heart rate, sweating, trouble sleeping, anxiety, heat intolerance, and fatigue. These symptoms are all fairly common for any pregnant woman. One way to determine whether the mother is hyperthyroid is that if she has Graves' disease, she will not usually gain a great deal of weight during pregnancy; she may even lose weight.

Graves' disease

Alice is a cousin of Stacy, Karen, Sarah, and Margaret – friends from earlier chapters. She is four weeks pregnant and notices that her heart is beating very fast all the time and she is also feeling very warm. She has lost a few pounds in weight, and her husband notices that her neck seems enlarged.

Alice and her husband go to their GP, who obtains thyroid blood tests to rule out hyperthyroidism. To her surprise, her doctor rules *in* the possibility of hyperthyroidism when results show that the free T4 level in Alice's blood is elevated while her TSH level is suppressed. The doctor immediately refers Alice to a thyroid specialist clinic where she is checked for thyroid-stimulating hormone receptor stimulating antibodies. The test result is very positive. Alice starts taking the antithyroid medication, propylthiouracil. Within three weeks, Alice begins to feel better. At six weeks, she is gaining weight and her heart has slowed noticeably. Alice is able to come off the propylthiouracil during the second half of her pregnancy, which proceeds normally. Her baby is checked carefully for hyperthyroidism, which fortunately, does not develop.

After the delivery, Alice again needs antithyroid medication, which she takes for a year. She does well.

Lab tests show that a hyperthyroid mother has high levels of free T4 and low levels of TSH. In this situation, a total T4 test (refer to Chapter 4) is not helpful at all, because the total T4 is always elevated in view of the increase in thyroid-binding globulin in the mother's system.

Hyperthyroidism needs to be controlled during pregnancy, otherwise it can lead to:

✔ Premature delivery

✔ Foetal malformations

✔ Low birth weight

✔ Hyperthyroidism in the infant

✔ High blood pressure and other problems in the mother

The development of hyperthyroidism during a pregnancy is relatively uncommon and is thought to affect around 1 in every 500 pregnancies.

This type of hyperthyroidism is associated with antibodies that stimulate the TSH receptors on thyroid cells and trigger the production of more thyroid hormone. In some cases, Graves' disease (refer to Chapter 6) occurs before pregnancy and reappears despite successful treatment with radioactive iodine, surgery, or antithyroid drugs. And, although mum may have normal thyroid function, she may still have antibodies that can pass through the placenta to the foetus, giving the foetus hyperthyroidism and a probable goitre.

Finding hyperthyroidism in the foetus

A number of signs suggest that the foetus has hyperthyroidism, most of which are determined during an ultrasound scan of the developing foetus. These signs include:

- ✔ Foetal goitre
- ✔ Very rapid foetal heart rate (over 160 beats per minute)
- ✔ Increased movement of the foetus
- ✔ Changes in foetal bones (increased bone maturity)
- ✔ Slowed foetal growth

If you are pregnant after successful treatment for Graves' disease, your foetus can become hyperthyroid because you still have thyroid-stimulating antibodies that can pass through the placenta. It's important for your doctor to monitor the foetus for signs of hyperthyroidism and check you for TSH receptor antibodies early in pregnancy. If your TSH receptor antibodies are elevated, but no signs of foetal hyperthyroidism is present, both are usually checked again after six months.

Treatment of hyperthyroidism in the foetus involves giving antithyroid drugs to the mother; the medication then passes through the placenta to decrease the thyroid function of the foetus. The mother may need to take thyroid hormone replacement as a result, however, because her thyroid function is reduced during the antithyroid treatment, as well.

The foetus may also show hyperthyroidism at birth if the mother has Graves' disease that is not well controlled or has a lot of TSH receptor stimulating antibodies. A mother who has a baby with neonatal hyperthyroidism is at especially high risk of having another in a subsequent pregnancy.

Hyperthyroidism in the newborn may not appear until the antithyroid drugs, obtained through the placenta, have cleared out of the baby's system. The baby will then have the usual signs of hyperthyroidism plus signs specific to a newborn, such as failure to thrive, increase in the yellow colour of the skin (jaundice due to increased bilirubin), and increased irritability. After the mother's thyroid-stimulating antibodies clear from the baby's blood, the baby will have normal thyroid function.

Treating the mother during pregnancy

Autoimmune hyperthyroidism tends to improve through the course of a pregnancy because of a general decline in the mother's autoimmunity. Other factors aiding the improvement of autoimmune hyperthyroidism include an increase in thyroxine-binding globulin, an increased loss of iodine in the urine, and an increase in TSH receptor blocking antibodies as the TSH receptor stimulating antibodies decline.

Radioactive iodine is not used to treat Graves' disease during a pregnancy, because the radiation can create malformations in the foetus and destroy the foetal thyroid gland.

The usual treatment for Graves' disease during pregnancy is the use of antithyroid drugs: propylthiouracil or carbimazole. The dose of antithyroid drug that is used is the least amount that can keep the free T4 in the upper part of the normal range (refer to Chapter 4 and Chapter 6). When this is done, the foetus receives the right amount of T4 from the mother.

A study of goitres in babies at birth found that 8 out of 11 were due to hypothyroidism in the baby, while 3 were due to hyperthyroidism. Of the 8 hypothyroid babies, 5 were due to excessive amounts of antithyroid drugs given to the mother during pregnancy. This evidence emphasises how important it is to give the least amount of antithyroid drug that allows the mother's thyroid function to return to normal.

A few circumstances require surgery rather than antithyroid drugs, including:

- ✔ Repeated failure to take antithyroid drugs.
- ✔ When the mother needs exceptionally high doses of medication.
- ✔ When a slow foetal heart rate suggests the foetus may have hypothyroidism due to the mother's antithyroid drug.
- ✔ The mother has extremely severe hyperthyroid symptoms.
- ✔ The mother experiences side effects, like a fall in white blood cells, from the drug.

If surgery is needed, the best time is between three and six months of pregnancy (second trimester), when it is least harmful to the foetus and the mother.

To prepare for surgery, the mother is sometimes given iodine. Iodine passes easily through the placenta to the foetus, where it can cause goitre and hypothyroidism. Iodine is also found in topical compounds and dyes used for better observation of the growing foetus. The use of iodine is necessary in these situations, but talk with your doctor about the consequences of excessive use.

Checking mother and child after birth

After a baby is born, a mother with Graves' disease can expect a worsening of her symptoms as her immune function increases and autoimmunity becomes severe again. Getting your thyroid function checked with blood tests after the delivery is important.

The easiest way to check the thyroid status of a newborn is to check the levels of free T4 and TSH in the umbilical cord blood. Treatment depends upon the findings.

Breastfeeding with Graves' disease

For many years, doctors believed that mothers who were being treated with antithyroid drugs for Graves' disease should not breastfeed because the drugs would enter her milk and pass to the baby. Recent studies have proved that this is not the case. You can breastfeed safely if you are taking antithyroid drugs for hyperthyroidism as long as the baby's development is closely monitored, and the lowest effective dose of drug is used.

Postpartum Graves' disease

Postpartum Graves' disease is not the same as postpartum thyroiditis (refer to Chapter 11). Graves' disease is associated with increased production of thyroid hormones due to stimulation by TSH receptor stimulating antibodies, whereas postpartum thyroiditis occurs when preformed thyroid hormone spills from a damaged thyroid. Treatment for these two conditions is therefore entirely different – postpartum Graves' disease is treated with anti-thyroid drugs, whereas postpartum thyroiditis, in which symptoms are usually mild, is treated with a beta-blocker if necessary. Postpartum thyroiditis is differentiated from Graves' disease by detecting a low uptake of injected technetium during a thyroid scan. Breast-feeding is usually only stopped for 30 hours after this investigation.

Postpartum thyroiditis is associated with thyroid autoantibodies. Some specialists recommend that all pregnant women have tests for thyroid autoantibodies early in pregnancy, as about 50 per cent of those with positive tests go on to develop postpartum thyroiditis.

Gestational transient thyrotoxicosis

Holly is a 27-year-old woman who is pregnant for the first time. She has a lot of morning sickness during the first few weeks of her pregnancy. She loses some weight, but believes this loss is due to the morning sickness. However, in the last few days, she notices other symptoms of a rapid heartbeat, fatigue, trouble sleeping, and a feeling of warmth all the time. She checks with her GP who suggests that Holly has Graves' disease. Thyroid function tests seem to confirm this and she is referred to a thyroid specialist clinic.

The doctor at the clinic notices that Holly's thyroid is not enlarged. He is concerned about the amount of vomiting that Holly describes and checks her for TSH receptor stimulating autoantibodies. The result is negative and Holly is told she probably has a condition called *gestational transient thyrotoxicosis* (GTT), which usually improves quickly. Holly takes a low dose of propranolol, a drug that relieves her symptoms, along with a drug for her vomiting. Over the next few weeks, Holly returns to normal and has no further trouble with hyperthyroid symptoms. Her thyroid function tests also return to normal.

Gestational transient thyrotoxicosis is actually more common than Graves' disease in pregnancy, occurring as often as two to three times in 100 pregnancies. Fortunately, GTT is generally mild. But sometimes the condition is more serious, and is occasionally confused with Graves' disease, leading to incorrect treatment.

GTT is due to the hormone called *human chorionic gonadotrophin* (HCG), which is produced by the placenta to maintain early pregnancy. HCG is at its highest level in the mother's circulation at around 10 weeks of pregnancy, but remains elevated throughout, and may appear in a form that is cleared very slowly from the mother's circulation. HCG can act as a thyroid stimulant, leading to increased free T4 and decreased TSH, which produces a diagnosis of hyperthyroidism. No TSH receptor stimulating antibodies are found in GTT.

About half of women with GTT show the typical symptoms of hyperthyroidism. In addition, many experience a significant increase in vomiting, sometimes called hyperemesis gravidarum. A goitre does not usually develop.

Most women with GTT need minimal treatment with a beta-blocker like propranolol (refer to Chapter 6). Sometimes, the mother is given fluids to replenish what she loses from vomiting. Occasionally, antithyroid drugs are needed for a short time, until levels of HCG begin to fall (usually after 10 weeks of pregnancy). However, in twin pregnancies, HCG levels may remain particularly high for a longer time period. Some studies have not shown a difference in the level of HCG between pregnant women who vomit a lot and those who do not. This evidence suggests that women who experience a lot of vomiting may make a form of HCG that is especially stimulating to the thyroid.

The most severe vomiting associated with GTT occurs when the level of thyroid hormone, the level of HCG, and the level of oestrogen in the pregnant mother are all at a maximum.

If you have symptoms of hyperthyroidism plus vomiting in early pregnancy, the likely diagnosis is GTT rather than Graves' disease. GTT usually improves after several weeks, while Graves' disease requires treatment throughout the pregnancy in many cases.

Hydatidiform mole and choriocarcinoma

Occasionally, as a result of some abnormality of the mother's egg or in fertilization, the placenta forms a series of grape-like clusters called a hydatidiform mole. No viable foetus develops from this mole, but in about 10 per cent of cases it can secrete large amounts of HCG and cause hyperthyroidism. The mother often experiences vaginal bleeding, and her uterus is not the correct size for the stage of the pregnancy (it's usually too large).

An ultrasound study in this situation shows the mole very clearly. Because no viable foetus is present, the pregnancy is terminated.

Very rarely – about 2 per cent of the time – the mole changes into a cancer called a choriocarcinoma, which can also make a large amount of HCG. Fortunately, this cancer is very treatable, and the patient can usually go on to have further children in the future.

Finding New Thyroid Nodules during Pregnancy

Because pregnant women have frequent exams, thyroid nodules are sometimes discovered during pregnancy. Treatment depends upon the tissue found in the nodule and the stage of the pregnancy.

The first step is to do a fine needle aspiration biopsy of the nodule (refer to Chapter 7). If the biopsy shows that a nodule is definitely cancer, and the patient is less than six months pregnant, she is usually offered thyroid surgery at that time. Between three and six months of pregnancy (second trimester) is the best time for this surgery because it offers the least chance of interfering with the development of the baby or of causing premature labour.

If the biopsy does not definitely show cancer, it is safe to wait until after the delivery, when a radioactive iodine scan is done (refer to Chapter 4). Keep in mind that after a radioactive iodine scan, the mother cannot breastfeed her baby. If the scan shows that the iodine uptake is high, the nodule probably isn't cancer. If the scan shows that the nodule remains cold, and the diagnosis remains uncertain, then surgery is needed to obtain a final diagnosis and determine the appropriate treatment. As radioactive iodine can remain in the body for several weeks, breastfeeding should be discontinued in nursing mothers.

If a scan is essential, an alternative is to use radioactive technetium. As technetium is cleared from the body within 30 hours, it is usually safe to continue breastfeeding after this time (discarding milk expressed in the 30 hours after receiving the radioactive injection), but seek advice from your physician.

Chapter 19

Developing Thyroid Conditions in Childhood

*N*ewborns and children with thyroid abnormalities present special problems because their brain and body are developing at the same time, and thyroid hormones are critical for their development. Thyroid hormones are needed in the right amount at the right time for a child to have normal mental function and normal growth.

Children can experience all the kinds of thyroid diseases that are seen in adults. This chapter discusses normal thyroid development and the impact of thyroid diseases on a developing human being. As a parent, you can do little to treat these conditions, but your early recognition of a problem, your understanding of the consequences if the problem is not treated, and your continued support of your child through treatment and recovery can help your child handle this challenge.

Understanding the Onset of Thyroid Function

First, a quick review. Thyroid hormones (T3 and T4) are produced when thyroid-stimulating hormone (TSH) stimulates the thyroid to make them. TSH is released from the pituitary gland when the hypothalamus produces thyrotrophin-releasing hormone (TRH). All these structures and their hormones are in place when a baby is born. Much recent research has established how this process comes about. (Refer to Chapter 3 for more on thyroid hormones and TSH.)

After just 15 weeks of development, the foetus shows function in its pituitary gland, and TRH can be detected. TSH and the other pituitary hormones start to appear between weeks 10 and 17. The thyroid is functioning by the 10th week, and its production of thyroid hormone becomes significant around the 20th week. The ability of thyroid hormone to shut off TSH production matures towards the end of the pregnancy and in the first two months after delivery.

The placenta acts as a barrier, preventing the mother's TSH from reaching the circulation of the foetus throughout the pregnancy. The placenta also contains an enzyme that breaks down the mother's thyroid hormones before they can reach the foetus. In breaking down the hormones, the enzyme releases iodine from the mother's hormones so the foetus can use the iodine to make thyroid hormone for itself. At the same time, the placenta is producing human chorionic gonadotrophin, a hormone that stimulates the thyroid (refer to Chapter 18).

As the pregnancy progresses, the enzyme in the placenta that breaks down the mother's thyroid hormones stops working as much, and other enzymes take over to convert T4 into the active hormone, T3. By not working so much, the placental enzyme no longer prevents the mother's T4 from getting to the foetus. This is very important, because the foetus needs the T4 for normal development, especially of its brain, at a time when it cannot make much T4 for itself.

One enzyme, which converts T4 to T3, works in the liver, the kidneys, and the thyroid. Another enzyme works mainly in the pituitary gland. If the foetus is not getting enough T4, the enzyme in the pituitary increases, and the other one decreases so the foetal brain gets enough T3.

When the baby is born, leaving the warmth of the uterus for the colder temperatures of the outside world, the baby's pituitary releases a large amount of TSH. This action stimulates the thyroid to release a large amount of T3 and T4, causing the temperature of the baby's body to rise. This process is known as the TSH surge. The TSH surge peaks after only 30 minutes but continues to stimulate extra thyroid hormone for the next 24 hours.

A premature baby has similar hormone changes to a normal-term baby, but to a lesser extent. It does not have as much of a TSH surge and does not produce as much thyroid hormone. The T3 does not increase as much either, because the converting enzymes are not yet as active. This baby cannot defend its body temperature in the way that a normal-term baby can.

As the baby grows, it stores more thyroid hormones in its thyroid along with thyroglobulin (refer to Chapter 4), and it produces more thyroid hormone.

The thyroid gland grows so the lobes are normally about the same size as the part of the baby's thumbs after the last joint (the terminal phalanx).

A lack of thyroid hormone during foetal growth has important consequences (refer to Chapter 12). Thyroid hormone is particularly important in the development of hearing, but many other body organs also need it for proper development. Some of the damage that results from lack of thyroid hormone includes the following:

- ✔ Immature bones
- ✔ Immature liver
- ✔ Reduced mental function
- ✔ Increased sleepiness

The brain is dependent on thyroid hormone for development for the first two to three years after birth. For every month that thyroid hormone is not given to a hypothyroid newborn, he or she suffers a loss of five IQ (intelligence quotient) points.

During the first 20 years of life, the free T3 and free T4 slowly decline, as does the total T3 and total T4 (check out Chapter 3 for an explanation of the difference between free and total). As oestrogen levels begin to rise during puberty in the female, her body makes more thyroid-binding globulin, and more total T3 and total T4. The decrease in the free T3 and free T4 is probably because of a gradual decline in TSH.

Screening the Newborn

Noah is the newborn son of Barry and Sally. Sally finds that Noah feeds poorly and is cold to the touch, but otherwise he appears fine.

As part of the UNITED KINGDOM neonatal screening programme, Noah is checked for hypothyroidism a few days after birth. The TSH level comes back high. The paediatrician notifies Barry and Sally and asks them to bring Noah in for testing. A blood test confirms that his TSH is elevated, and the free T4 is low. The paediatrician diagnoses congenital hypothyroidism.

Noah has a thyroid scan which shows little active thyroid tissue. Noah is given thyroid hormone, and his feeding and his body temperature rapidly improve. Sally notices that Noah looks less puffy as well. The doctor measures thyroid functions frequently until Noah stabilises. Noah grows and feeds normally. He does not appear to have any problems reaching his developmental milestones. The major reason for screening newborns for thyroid disease is to diagnose congenital hypothyroidism as early as possible. Congenital hypothyroidism means hypothyroidism that is present when the baby is born (see the next section, 'Coping with Hypothyroidism in Children').

In a study of 800 children with congenital hypothyroidism before the era of screening, the average IQ was 80, which is low. However, those babies with obvious signs of hypothyroidism who had received testing and appropriate treatment had a normal IQ. Because the consequence of not treating hypothyroidism in newborns is so great and the response to early treatment is so successful, screening for thyroid disease is considered essential.

Screening is a simple process. A spot of the baby's blood, from a heel prick, is placed on filter paper. Then the filter paper is tested for TSH. If the TSH is very high, the baby has a regular blood test for TSH and free T4, and the doctor begins treating the baby with thyroid hormone while waiting for the result. If the TSH is moderately raised, blood tests are taken, but no treatment is begun until the diagnosis is confirmed. The reason is that up to 75 per cent of babies with a TSH that is moderately raised during the screening test will have normal thyroid function according to the regular blood test. This is because a TSH surge occurs immediately after birth, and screening on the first day may result in a false diagnosis due to this surge.

The screening test is not perfect. Children with secondary hypothyroidism, which results from the body's failure to secrete TSH, are missed. And screening does not identify children with a normal TSH and a low T4 whose TSH becomes abnormal a week later. Premature babies, especially, may show this pattern. Babies who fail to secrete TSH often have failure of other hormones as well, which leads to many signs and symptoms that point to ill-health.

Infants with low birth weight are sometimes misdiagnosed because they tend to have low levels of hormones at birth, which soon rise to normal.

Congenital hypothyroidism affects about 1 in 3,750 babies. Screening of newborns for hypothyroidism is now carried out by law in most westernised countries, and a major campaign is underway to promote neonatal screening for thyroid disease throughout the world.

Coping with Hypothyroidism in Children

A number of conditions can cause hypothyroidism in newborn and older children. Specialists disagree as to whether pregnant mothers should have routine testing for hypothyroidism to protect their babies from a hypothyroid environment. A study in the *New England Journal of Medicine* shows that babies experience a slight loss of IQ if their mothers are hypothyroid and untreated during pregnancy.

Transient congenital hypothyroidism

Some babies are diagnosed with hypothyroidism at birth because their TSH levels are high, but these levels fall to normal shortly after birth. This condition is called transient congenital hypothyroidism because it doesn't last. One common cause of this condition is iodine deficiency in the mother (refer to Chapter 12).

This condition is especially prevalent in very low-birth-weight infants, who are normally screened for thyroid disease not only at birth, but also at two weeks and six weeks of age.

Because this condition is so common in premature infants, the question is whether these babies need thyroid supplementation for a short time at birth. A study in the *Texas Medical Journal* in 2000, suggests that babies who have gestated for more than 27 weeks at the time of birth don't need supplemental thyroid hormone and may actually do worse with such treatment, whereas babies who spend less than 27 weeks in the womb may benefit from supplementation.

Sometimes, determining whether hypothyroidism is transient or permanent isn't possible. In this case, the baby is treated with thyroid hormone until the age of 4 years, and then treatment is stopped for a short time to see if the child can make his or her own thyroid hormone. This treatment does not affect the child's brain development.

Congenital hypothyroidism

Babies who are born with hypothyroidism that doesn't correct itself shortly after birth have congenital hypothyroidism. Thanks to neonatal thyroid screening, this condition is no longer a significant cause of mental retardation.

Causes

There are many causes of congenital hypothyroidism, but 80 per cent of cases result from *thyroid dysgenesis* – a failure of the thyroid gland to grow or to end up in its proper place in the neck. Thyroid dysgenesis can result in:

- No thyroid at all (a condition called *thyroid agenesis*)
- A small gland that makes little thyroid hormone (*thyroid hypoplasia*)
- A thyroid gland that grows in the wrong place, often at the base of the tongue (*ectopic thyroid*)

Some other, less frequent causes of congenital hypothyroidism include:

- An inability of a baby's thyroid to respond to TSH.
- Exposure of the mother to radioactive iodine that destroys the baby's thyroid.
- Failure of the baby's hypothalamus to release TRH (thyrotrophin-releasing hormone) – a condition called *hypothalamic hypothyroidism*.
- An abnormality of some step in the synthesis of thyroid hormone.

With the exception of maternal exposure to radioactive iodine, these conditions are all relatively rare genetic diseases (see Chapter 17).

Signs and symptoms

Many babies with congenital hypothyroidism have few signs or symptoms of hypothyroidism at birth. This condition is discovered by screening (refer to the section 'Screening the Newborn' earlier in the chapter). If the condition is severe, the baby shows some or all of the following signs:

- Low body temperature
- Slow heart rate
- Poor feeding
- Umbilical hernia (an outward protrusion of the umbilicus – the belly button – that may contain intestines)

Once the condition is recognised and confirmed, treatment is started immediately. A thyroid scan just before treating the baby may help detect any functioning thyroid tissue, a lack of which indicates the need for lifelong treatment. If no tissue is seen on the thyroid scan, a thyroid ultrasound shows whether tissue exists and whether it's unable to take up iodine, possibly due to a genetic abnormality. This information is helpful in counselling the parents about the chance of hypothyroidism in future children.

Treatment

Babies with congenital hypothyroidism usually receive a relatively high dose of thyroxine (T4) hormone replacement for the first week to restore their thyroid hormone levels. The daily dose given afterwards depends on their individual needs.

The baby's thyroid function is usually checked at 7, 14, and 28 days. In view of all the changes taking place in thyroid function soon after birth, the stabilisation of thyroid function may take time. Once the tests are normal and stable, they are typically measured every three months until two years of age and then every year.

Proper dosing of thyroid hormone is determined by thyroid-function tests and by ensuring that the baby is growing properly. The height and weight of the baby are checked regularly to verify the hormone dosage.

If thyroid hormone treatment is delayed more than four to eight weeks after birth, a child with congenital hypothyroidism will almost certainly have some decrease in intellectual function.

Acquired hypothyroidism

Children may acquire hypothyroidism at any time after birth. When hypothyroidism occurs in a child over the age of two, it does not damage brain function, but it does greatly affect growth and development.

Causes

Children may develop hypothyroidism for all the same reasons as adults. Iodine deficiency is, by far, the most common cause throughout the world. Where iodine is sufficient, autoimmune thyroiditis (check out Chapter 5) is the leading cause. Less common reasons for acquired hypothyroidism include:

- Drugs like iodine or lithium
- Irradiation – externally (for a tumour, for example) or internally, in treatment of hyperthyroidism with radioactive iodine
- Removal of the thyroid for any reason
- Abnormal production of thyroid hormone
- Resistance to thyroid hormone
- Central or secondary hypothyroidism due to a tumour in the pituitary or hypothalamus or a lack of production of TSH or TRH

Signs and symptoms

Again, the findings in these conditions are similar to the signs and symptoms found in adults, except that a growing, developing child experiences the consequences of poor growth. Constipation and dry skin are a feature of any hypothyroid person. In addition, children do not keep pace with normal height and weight charts.

A child who becomes hypothyroid after he or she starts school has trouble with schoolwork and keeping up with their friends' level of physical activity due to lack of energy.

Interestingly, some of these kids appear unusually muscular, despite their weakness, as they develop swelling of muscle fibres – a condition called *muscle pseudohypertrophy*.

The growth of the skeleton and the teeth is delayed, and other signs include:

- ✔ Enlarged thyroid (goitre), unless it is previously removed
- ✔ Dry, cool skin that is puffy, pale, and yellowish
- ✔ Brittle nails and dry, brittle hair that tends to fall out excessively
- ✔ Swelling that does not retain an indentation, especially of the legs
- ✔ Hoarseness and slow speech with a thickened tongue
- ✔ An expressionless face
- ✔ A slow pulse

Some of these children occasionally show early sexual development. This development is thought to result from their high levels of TSH, which has a similar structure to follicle-stimulating hormone (FSH). As a result, TSH activates cells that normally respond to FSH, so girls may have early vaginal bleeding, and boys may have large testicles for their age. Boys do not have a lot of male hormone (testosterone) however, as its production results from the action of another hormone, luteinizing hormone (LH). TSH does not share features with LH. The girls, however, do have increased oestrogen for their age since their ovaries can respond to the FSH-like properties of TSH; LH-like stimulation is not needed for this.

Adolescents who develop hypothyroidism have signs and symptoms similar to those found in an adult, with a few differences. If the child has begun puberty, further sexual development may stop unless the child is given thyroid hormone treatment. The growth of permanent teeth is often delayed, and the child doesn't gain height as quickly as expected.

When a lack of TRH or TSH is the cause, the signs and symptoms of hypothyroidism are usually milder. The main symptoms are due to the underlying cause, such as a brain tumour, for example, in which the child complains of headaches or trouble with vision.

Laboratory confirmation

A TSH and free T4 test can confirm the diagnosis of hypothyroidism. In order to make a diagnosis of chronic (autoimmune) thyroiditis, the child is tested for the presence of thyroid autoantibodies. The child's bone age is determined with X-rays to evaluate any growth abnormalities.

If central hypothyroidism is responsible, the free T4 and the TSH are low, as are other hormones made in the pituitary gland. An X-ray or scan of the pituitary is then needed to look for a tumour.

Treatment

The current treatment for hypothyroidism is thyroxine (T4) hormone replacement. However, some studies in adults have been given both T3 and T4 replacement, in the same proportions that are made in the normal thyroid and this approach may gain future support (see Chapter 5).

In most cases, the dose of replacement hormone is adjusted until the TSH is normal. However, if the cause is central hypothyroidism, TSH is not used as a guide because the pituitary is not making any TSH.

In some cases, starting the child at a low dose and gradually increasing to the full therapeutic dose is necessary. Some children show more symptoms when they suddenly go from no thyroid hormone to full replacement. They experience trouble sleeping, restlessness, and deterioration in their school performance. Rarely, headaches may develop due to increased pressure in the brain. Lowering the dose and gradually building it back up helps this situation.

If the child's growth is delayed, he or she usually catches up when thyroid hormone is given.

Giving too much thyroid hormone may cause early closure of bone growth resulting in stunted growth and a decrease in bone mineral content.

Dealing with Hyperthyroidism in Children

Hyperthyroidism is rarely seen in babies and is less common in children and adolescents than it is in adults. Almost always, kids with hyperthyroidism have Graves' disease (refer to Chapter 6). When a newborn is hyperthyroid, usually the mother is also hyperthyroid (check out Chapter 18), and the mother's thyroid-stimulating antibodies have passed to the foetus. When these antibodies naturally clear from the foetus after it's born, the hyperthyroidism subsides about 3 to 12 weeks after birth.

Signs and symptoms

When a mother with hyperthyroidism passes a large amount of thyroid-stimulating antibodies to her baby through the placenta, the foetus develops hyperthyroidism. The signs of the hyperthyroidism in the foetus include:

- ✔ Rapid heart rate

- ✔ Increased foetal movements

- ✔ Poor foetal body growth

- ✔ Abnormally rapid bone growth

After the baby is born, the baby shows a number of signs and symptoms of hyperthyroidism. They are the result of excessive metabolism and include:

- ✔ Low birth weight and failure to gain weight

- ✔ Increased appetite

- ✔ Irritability

- ✔ Rapid heart rate

- ✔ Enlarged thyroid

- ✔ Prominent eyes

Hyperthyroidism is rare in children under the age of five and is usually due to Graves' disease. Once in a while, the cause is a functioning *thyroid adenoma* – a new growth of tissue on or within the thyroid that makes excessive amounts of thyroid hormone. Girls develop thyroid adenomas more often than boys. A family history of other autoimmune diseases (for example, Type 1 diabetes) is often present when the cause is Graves' disease.

In children under the age of five, the signs and symptoms of hyperthyroidism are like those seen in adults (refer to Chapter 6) plus problems resulting from the needs of a growing child who has now reached school age. Unique signs at this age include:

- ✔ Poor school performance

- ✔ Trouble sleeping

- ✔ Poor athletic performance related to muscle weakness

- ✔ Tiredness

- ✔ More rapid growth in height but early closure of bone growth

- ✔ Stunted final height

- ✔ Irritability

These children are hungry all the time but don't gain weight despite eating. They generally have mild eye disease. They have a goitre and also have bowel movements more frequently than normal.

Laboratory confirmation

Confirmation of the diagnosis of hyperthyroidism is made from a free T4 and a TSH level. If foetal hyperthyroidism is suspected, these levels are determined from umbilical cord blood at birth. If hyperthyroidism is present, the free T4 is high and the TSH low. Rarely, if the hyperthyroidism is due to excessive TSH secretion from the pituitary, the TSH is high. In that case, the baby is screened for a pituitary tumour.

Treatment

If your child has hyperthyroidism, there are many treatment options. The important thing to remember is that continued vigilance is needed, as all forms of treatment are associated with the recurrence of hyperthyroidism or the development of hypothyroidism in some cases.

You need to ensure that your child's condition is followed up regularly after treatment because the disease process is ongoing. Regularly means every six months or yearly, as recommended by your doctor. All children with neonatal thyrotoxicosis usually have yearly neurological assessments until at least the age of six years.

If a developing foetus is hyperthyroid, antithyroid drugs are given to the mother. The drugs pass through the placenta to affect the foetus's thyroid hormone production. The goal is to have a foetal heart rate less than 140 beats per minute. Sometimes, the mother takes a beta-blocker (such as propranolol) to control severe symptoms.

Treatment of hyperthyroidism in babies also involves antithyroid drugs. Once treatment is given, the baby rapidly improves. In a few months, the antithyroid drugs are withdrawn as the thyroid-stimulating antibodies passed from mother to baby naturally disappear from the baby's circulation.

Radioactive iodine

At one time, doctors resisted using radioactive iodine to treat hyperthyroidism in children. However, this treatment is more commonly used today because long-term studies show no negative effects upon the child. Specifically, no increase in cancer or loss of fertility and no negative effect upon the offspring of children treated with radioactive iodine is found.

The problem with radioactive iodine is that most children become hypothyroid after some time. (The same is true of adults; refer to Chapter 6.) In addition, thyroid eye disease may get worse when radioactive iodine is used because of the release of a lot of antigen (material that the immune system may recognise as foreign) from the thyroid.

Antithyroid drugs

Antithyroid drugs such as propylthiouracil (PTU) and carbimazole are the preferred treatment for hyperthyroidism in children. They take three to six weeks to work, but they control the disease in at least 85 per cent of children. If the medication doesn't work, the child usually has a very large goitre or doesn't take the medication as prescribed. In most cases, treatment is continued for two to four years.

How does the doctor choose which of these two drugs to use? PTU has the advantage of blocking the conversion of T4 to T3, whereas carbimazole lasts longer after taking it. In practise, these differences don't seem to matter much.

If the disease is going to recur after the pills are stopped, the child usually has measurable amounts of TSH receptor-stimulating antibodies. This test is done at the time treatment is stopped to help predict a future recurrence. The drugs fail to produce a permanent remission in up to half of children treated, even though 85 per cent are controlled.

Just as in adults, antithyroid medications cause side effects in children. The most important is that the production of white blood cells is halted. The prescribing doctor monitors white blood cells, and if the white cell count falls, the drug is stopped. If PTU was used initially, the child is not switched to carbimazole or vice versa – a totally different treatment is needed. Sometimes, the white cell count falls a little, but it returns to normal after some weeks. Another important side effect is the development of a rash, which is treated without needing to stop taking the drug.

If your child is taking an antithyroid drug, you need to promptly report symptoms or signs of infection, especially a sore throat.

Surgery of the thyroid

Sometimes, antithyroid drugs cause serious side effects or the child doesn't take the pills correctly, and radioactive iodine is unsuitable (usually because the parents are concerned about giving radioactivity to their child). In these cases, surgery is a safe and rapid form of treatment in the hands of a competent surgeon who has experience with children. If possible, the child should have normal thyroid function accomplished with antithyroid drugs before having surgery. Iodine is given for two weeks prior to surgery to block the thyroid gland and reduce blood flow into it. The usual operation is a near total thyroidectomy (check out Chapter 13 for more on surgery of the thyroid).

Sometimes, the surgeon can leave enough thyroid tissue to retain thyroid function while eliminating hyperthyroidism, but the child is checked at least every six months to a year to detect recurrence or loss of thyroid function and the need for thyroid medication.

Diagnosing Goitres in Children

An enlarged thyroid gland is actually the most common thyroid abnormality found in children. It occurs in about 5 per cent of all children. A child with an enlarged thyroid usually has normal thyroid function.

The most common cause of thyroid enlargement in children is autoimmune thyroiditis (refer to Chapter 5). The second most common cause is a multinodular goitre (refer to Chapter 9).

Telling these causes apart is important because autoimmune thyroiditis can lead to hypothyroidism (or sometimes hyperthyroidism), whereas multinodular goitre does not. Obtaining thyroid autoantibody studies can tell the difference, pointing to autoimmune thyroiditis if the results are positive. Testing the child's levels of free T4 and TSH verifies whether his or her thyroid function is normal.

These goitres sometimes get smaller and then larger again, sometimes growing at different rates in different parts of the thyroid, leading to a multinodular thyroid gland.

Treatment is given if the large thyroid is pressing on nearby structures like the oesophagus and trachea, or is disfiguring. The treatment is either surgery or radioactive iodine. The thyroid is checked every six months for a few visits, then yearly.

If the goitre is painful, the diagnosis is more likely subacute or acute thyroiditis (refer to Chapter 11). These diseases cause similar signs and symptoms in children as they cause in adults. Subacute thyroiditis generally makes a child less sick than acute thyroiditis. Subacute thyroiditis affects the whole gland, whereas acute thyroiditis may swell only part of the gland. If acute thyroiditis occurs several times, this occurrence can be due to a malformation in the thyroid that requires surgery to correct it.

Linking Nodules and Cancer in Children

Children rarely get thyroid nodules, but when they do, the nodules indicate cancer more frequently than they do in adults. The signs that make a nodule particularly suspicious for cancer are the same as in adults:

- Rapid growth
- Painlessness

> ✔ Firmness and fixation
>
> ✔ Nodes felt in the neck

While a functioning nodule or a cystic nodule (refer to Chapter 7) is rarely cancerous in an adult, this case isn't true in children.

A very important clue that a child's nodule is cancerous is past exposure to irradiation. Exposure leads to nodules and cancer in multiple places in the thyroid. (The leading type of thyroid cancer in both children and adults is papillary – the type of cancer most closely associated with irradiation exposure.)

A fine needle biopsy of the nodule is carried out if the doctor suspects cancer, but this test isn't as helpful in children as it is in adults. A 1996 study in the *Journal of Pediatric Surgery* shows that a correct diagnosis of thyroid cancer is made in only 3 of 7 biopsies. It's not clear why this result is so – perhaps because a child's nodule is small and easily missed by the needle.

Children tend to have more cancer spread into the neck and into the lungs at the time they are diagnosed than adults, but this fact does not make their prognosis worse. The cancer is managed just like adult cancer with a total thyroidectomy (refer to Chapter 13), preserving the parathyroid glands and the recurrent laryngeal nerves. This surgery is followed with radioactive destruction of the remaining thyroid tissue. The patient is placed on thyroid hormone to replace the thyroid and to suppress growth of new thyroid tissue.

Children with thyroid cancer are monitored with thyroglobulin blood tests; this test should read close to 0 shortly after surgery. The blood tests are carried out every six months to a year. If the level of thyroglobulin rises, a whole body scan is needed to look for any tissue that takes up iodine. The scan may use new recombinant TSH (refer to Chapter 14) so the patient does not have to stop taking thyroid hormone to perform this study. If all the iodine is found in the neck, local surgery is often enough to eliminate the additional thyroid cancer tissue. If the tissue is spread around the body, a large dose of radioactive iodine destroys it.

Chapter 20

Maturing: Thyroid Disease in Later Life

....

In This Chapter

▶ Discovering how many older people have thyroid disease

▶ Recognising the difficulty of diagnosis

▶ Dealing with hypo- and hyperthyroidism

▶ Treating thyroid nodules in older people

....

*B*efore talking thyroids, you need to know that 'older people' are those aged 65 or older. Not that far away! And most people over that age still feel young thanks to the knock-on effects of the fact that 50 is undoubtedly the new 40. Compared with just a few generations ago, modern people in later life are usually more outgoing, active, and generally more youthful.

Even so, older people are often afflicted with thyroid disease – a diagnosis that's often missed for two key reasons. First, when an older person goes to a doctor, hospital, or nursing home, the illness or condition that prompts him or her to seek care is, naturally, the doctor's primary focus. Secondly, symptoms of thyroid disease often mirror symptoms of other conditions so, even if the doctor looks for these other conditions, thyroid disease itself is often overlooked.

When doctors are taught about disease, they learn a set of signs and symptoms that are characteristic of each particular illness. Unfortunately, older people with thyroid disease may have no typical symptoms, and when they do occur, their symptoms are often the opposite of those expected. The only way doctors are going to discover thyroid disease in many older people is with screening – obtaining thyroid function tests from a person who appears healthy – but this step is controversial.

Screening for thyroid disease in older people has its own problems, as screening picks up a lot of subclinical disease – a situation where one blood test is not normal but another is, and the patient is otherwise well. There's tremendous controversy concerning what to do with subclinical thyroid disease. As a community, doctors haven't yet made any final decisions about whether to treat subclinical thyroid disease, wait for symptoms to develop, or wait for both thyroid blood tests to become abnormal.

Assessing the Extent of the Problem

To determine how many older people have thyroid disease, doctors need to decide what 'thyroid disease' actually means. Is having an abnormal TSH level sufficient to make a diagnosis, or is an abnormal free T4 level needed as well? (Check out Chapter 4 for information about these tests.) This question is difficult to answer in older people because they often have so many symptoms, many of which relate to other conditions. Some doctors consider an abnormal TSH is insufficient evidence of thyroid disease, and use the term *subclinical* to describe the situation where the TSH is abnormal but the free T4 is normal. Some doctors do not support treating a patient with subclinical thyroid disease. Yet many studies show that treatment reduces or eliminates many of the symptoms. On the other hand, treating an older person, particularly with thyroid hormone for hypothyroidism, is not always helpful, as this chapter discusses later.

In one study from the United Kingdom, published in the *Archives of Internal Medicine* in January 2001, all patients age 65 or older were tested for thyroid disease when entering hospital. Out of 280 patients (leaving out those with known thyroid disease), 9 had hypothyroidism and 5 had hyperthyroidism that was not previously suspected. An additional 21 people had subclinical hypothyroidism (high TSH, normal free T4), and 12 had subclinical hyperthyroidism (low TSH, normal free T4). Overall, nearly 40 per cent of the older people not thought to have thyroid disease had some evidence of it. Do all these people need treatment?

Writing in rebuttal to this study, other authors suggest that many older people with subclinical disease actually have temporary abnormalities due to other conditions.

In another study of older people not in hospital, unsuspected hyperthyroidism was discovered in 1 per cent, and unsuspected hypothyroidism was discovered in 2 per cent. So, 3 of 100 older people are walking around with clinical thyroid disease. This figure may not seem like a lot, but in the population of the United Kingdom, where 16 per cent of the population are aged 65 and over, this fact means that more than 290,000 older people are walking around with undetected and highly treatable thyroid disease. (That number does not even account for the age group 35 to 65, which contains many more cases of undiagnosed thyroid disease.)

Large population studies have shown that 10 per cent of women over age 65 have elevated TSH levels. Most of them do not have symptoms of thyroid disease. Isn't it interesting that there's no argument about screening babies for thyroid disease (when the occurrence of abnormal tests is 1 in 3,750), yet the debate continues about screening older people (when 3 in 100 cases of clinical thyroid disease are likely)?

Some doctors believe that everyone should have screening for thyroid disease beginning at age 35 and every five years thereafter. Unfortunately, costs get in the way, even though screening is easily done with a TSH test. If this test is abnormal, then a free T4 test is done. If both tests are abnormal, the patient is treated for thyroid disease. If only the TSH is abnormal, it's reasonable to take a careful history and do a physical examination, and then decide on treatment based upon that evaluation.

Understanding Sources of Confusion in Diagnosis

The natural consequences of ageing, the many complicating diseases found in older people, and the effects of medication can all confuse a diagnosis of thyroid disease. In fact, ageing and other diseases can cause symptoms that are identical to those found in thyroid disease. Medications can also affect laboratory tests to confuse the diagnosis even further (refer to Chapter 10). Diagnosing thyroid problems in older people therefore requires the detective work of a medical Sherlock Holmes.

Acknowledging other diseases

Certain diseases that affect thyroid test results are found more often in older than in younger people making the outcome appear as if a person has thyroid disease when they do not. The most common confusing factors in thyroid testing are

- Poor nutrition
- Poorly controlled diabetes
- Liver disease
- Heart failure

Any severe illness can also cause a temporary fall in T4 that is sometimes misdiagnosed as hypothyroidism.

Taking medications

Drugs often taken in later life that can alter thyroid function tests include the following:

- ✔ Epilepsy drugs, such as carbamazepine and phenytoin, cause the rapid breakdown of thyroid hormones in the liver which, in turn, lowers thyroid hormone levels in the blood.

- ✔ Aspirin decreases the binding of thyroid hormones to thyroid-binding globulin, which lowers the total (but not the free) T4.

- ✔ Corticosteroid drugs, such as prednisone, decrease thyroxine-binding globulin levels.

- ✔ Drugs for abnormal heart rhythm, particularly amiodarone, can cause both hypothyroidism and hyperthyroidism.

- ✔ Heparin, used for anticoagulation, can cause a temporary rise in T4 as it displaces it from binding proteins.

Discovering Hypothyroidism in Older People

Victor is a 68-year-old man who is feeling a bit fatigued. He has put on a few pounds, and feels cold when others seem comfortable. He also notices that he is more constipated than before. Victor thinks all these changes are the natural effects of ageing. Although he doesn't like to talk about it, his constipation is now a serious problem, and this symptom is what brings him to his doctor. The doctor observes that Victor's pulse is slow and that his eyebrows and eyelashes are rather sparse. He tells Victor that he believes this fact is due to hypothyroidism and sends him for thyroid function tests.

The TSH level comes back high at 9 µU/ml (microunits per millilitre), but his free T4 is within the normal range. Because his doctor is unsure of what to do, he refers him to a specialist who tells Victor that he appears to have subclinical hypothyroidism, although he thinks the symptoms Victor describes are due to his thyroid, so it's not really subclinical at all. He puts Victor on thyroid hormone replacement pills.

After two weeks, Victor notices with relief that his bowel movements improve. He feels less tired and much less cold. Repeat thyroid function tests show his TSH is now 6 μU/ml (microunits per millilitre), which is still a little high, so his dose of thyroid hormone is increased. A month later, his TSH test is down in the normal range, and Victor states that he is now back to his normal, mildly constipated self.

Deciphering signs and symptoms

The diagnosis of hypothyroidism is so easily missed in the elderly because so many of the changes our bodies experience as we grow older are typical findings in hypothyroidism. Some of the most important include:

✔ Slowing of mental function

✔ Slowing of physical function

✔ Tendency to have a lower body temperature

✔ Intolerance of cold

✔ Constipation

✔ Hardening of the arteries

✔ Elevation of blood fats (especially 'bad' LDL-cholesterol)

✔ Weight gain

✔ Elevation of blood pressure

✔ Anaemia

✔ Muscle cramps

✔ Dry skin

✔ Hair loss

All the above changes are common effects of ageing but are also signs and symptoms of hypothyroidism.

On the other hand, some signs found in older people tend to point away from a diagnosis of hypothyroidism, making an accurate diagnosis even less likely. For example, older people get Parkinson's disease, which results in tremors, or they simply develop senile tremors. Many elderly people lose weight because of poor nutrition; they may also develop anxiety and nervousness. These symptoms definitely don't neatly fit into the list of symptoms of hypothyroidism and may even point to an overactive thyroid gland, even though their thyroid is functioning below par. In addition, many elderly persons with hypothyroidism do not develop a goitre.

Getting laboratory confirmation

The only way to know for sure that an older person does not have hypothyroidism is to obtain thyroid function tests. If hypothyroidism is present, the free T4 is low and the TSH is high (refer to Chapter 4). Often the TSH is high but the free T4 is normal – the situation known as subclinical hypothyroidism. The only way to determine whether hypothyroidism is having an effect upon the patient is to give a trial of thyroid hormone, although, the patient does not always feel much different on medication.

Trying thyroid hormone for subclinical patients

Among older people with subclinical thyroid disease and a TSH level of less than 10, only half show some clinical improvement after receiving thyroxine (T4 hormone replacement). Such patients should probably not have treatment if they complain of angina heart pain. Most people whose TSH level is over 20 µU/ml (microunits per millilitre) tend to improve with treatment, however.

An important study, whose results indicate that subclinical hypothyroidism in older people is worth treating, was published in *Clinical Endocrinology* in 2000. In this study of 1,843 people aged 55 and over, those with an elevated TSH but a normal free T4 had a three times greater risk of developing dementia and Alzheimer's disease than those with normal TSH and free T4 – even when followed for as short a time as just two years. Concluding that the lower the free T4 (though still in the normal range), the higher the incidence of dementia and Alzheimer's. Those individuals with positive antiperoxidase antibodies (refer to Chapter 4) also had a higher incidence of dementia. This report is the first study to suggest that subclinical hypothyroidism in older people increases their risk of dementia and Alzheimer's disease.

Another factor that influences treatment decisions is that an older patient who has subclinical hypothyroidism along with another autoimmune disorder – such as Type 1 diabetes, pernicious anaemia, rheumatoid arthritis, or premature greying of the hair – is likely to eventually develop clinical hypothyroidism.

If you have subclinical thyroid disease and your doctor starts you on thyroid hormone replacement, there are several reasons why you may want to continue that treatment. If you test positive for thyroid autoantibodies and you have a high TSH, chances are very good that you'll develop clinical hypothyroidism in the future. Also, your cholesterol level may benefit from the thyroid hormone; a measurement of cholesterol before and after taking the pills often shows that it is lowered significantly. Thyroid hormone also lowers a chemical in the blood called *homocysteine*, which if raised, is now known to contribute to heart disease.

Taking treatment slowly

As far as treatment is concerned, it's important that the doctor goes slowly (which is, of course, against their usual nature). Treatment ideally starts with a very low dose of thyroxine (for example, 25 micrograms), increasing every four to six weeks until the TSH is at the upper limit of normal. You do not want excessive treatment as this increase sometimes worsens heart pain and increases shortness of breath, palpitations, and rapid heartbeats, as well as nervousness and heat intolerance. Even the first exposure to a small dose of thyroxine may bring on angina chest pain. A dose that is excessive can also lead to osteoporosis (brittle bones).

The major problem doctors have when treating older people with hypothyroidism is often compliance – ensuring that someone remembers to take his or her medication. Putting the pills into a case with daily slots may help.

Testing thyroid function on a regular basis to ensure that the TSH and free T4 levels remain normal is also important. Testing every six months is usually adequate.

Managing Hyperthyroidism in Older People

ANECDOTE

Toni is the 76-year-old aunt of Stacy and Karen (refer to Chapter 5 for more on them). Her husband notices that she seems depressed lately. While she used to love cooking, she seems to have lost interest. She sits on her couch most of the day, doing much of anything. She gains several pounds in weight and seems fatigued most of the time. Toni's doctor suggests that perhaps she is hypothyroid. He obtains thyroid function tests and, to his surprise, the free T4 is elevated and the TSH is suppressed, suggesting a diagnosis of hyperthyroidism. He sends Toni to the local thyroid specialist clinic.

The clinic finds that Toni does not have a goitre. However, her pulse is somewhat fast. The doctor makes a diagnosis of apathetic hyperthyroidism and explains to Toni's husband that this type of hyperthyroidism is not uncommon in older people. He starts Toni on the antithyroid drug, carbimazole. After six weeks, Toni's thyroid function tests are normal. The carbimazole is stopped and Toni is given radioactive iodine several days later.

Toni is feeling so much better that she invites the entire family to a delicious buffet in a lovely dining room recently remodelled by Toni's husband, where they all chat about their various thyroid problems.

Sorting through confusing signs and symptoms

Hyperthyroidism is less common than hypothyroidism, but it's still a significant problem among the elderly. As with hypothyroidism, the symptoms of an overactive thyroid are easily confused with the normal signs of ageing. The following characteristics are among the similarities between normal ageing and hyperthyroidism, and the person often experiences:

✔ Shaking

✔ Weight loss

✔ Irregular heart rhythm

✔ Increased threat of congestive heart failure

✔ Intolerance to heat

✔ Profuse sweating

✔ Fatigue and weakness

At the same time, older people may develop signs that aren't consistent with hyperthyroidism at all. They may appear entirely apathetic, sitting very quietly, acting depressed, and showing fatigue and weight gain. This combination is the picture of apathetic hyperthyroidism that Toni experiences. In addition, many older patients with hyperthyroidism don't have a goitre.

Sometimes, the only sign of hyperthyroidism is the finding of *atrial fibrillation*, a rapid and irregular heartbeat. (If you're diagnosed with atrial fibrillation, you usually need to take an anticoagulant to prevent blood clots forming in the irregularly beating heart. After the heart rhythm is restored to normal, the anti-coagulant is stopped.)

If your heart rhythm suddenly becomes very irregular, and your doctor tells you that it's atrial fibrillation, ask your doctor to remember to check your thyroid function tests.

Loss of bone is another important consequence of hyperthyroidism. Older people, particularly women whose bones are naturally thinner, cannot afford to lose more bone. One study, published in the *Journal of Clinical Investigation* in 2000, shows that older people with hyperthyroidism have significant reduction in bone density when compared to a similar group of people without hyperthyroidism. After people with hyperthyroidism are successfully treated, however, their bone mineral density improves within six months. Other studies show a definite increase in bone fracture risk in people with hyperthyroidism.

Securing a diagnosis

Thyroid function tests remain the key method for diagnosing hyperthyroidism in older people. If hyperthyroidism is present, the free T4 is high and the TSH is suppressed. Occasionally, the T4 is normal but the free T3 is elevated, a condition called *T3 thyrotoxicosis* (check out Chapter 6). This condition is especially common if a hyperactive nodule is the source of the hyperthyroidism.

The treatment of choice for hyperthyroidism in the elderly is radioactive iodine (RAI). With a single treatment, the disease is brought under control in four to six weeks. RAI avoids the problems associated with taking daily anti-thyroid pills. However, many people who take RAI develop hypothyroidism and then need a daily thyroid hormone pill for the rest of their lives.

A beta-blocker such as propranolol is also useful in controlling symptoms of hyperthyroidism (such as tremor, nervousness, sweating, and rapid heart rate).

If RAI is given to treat a hyperactive thyroid, there is occasionally a sudden release of thyroid hormones as the thyroid tissues break down. In an older person, this reaction can lead to a sudden worsening of heart failure and a very rapid heart rate, as well as chest pain. To avoid this complication, antithyroid drugs are given for six weeks before the RAI is given. When someone has normal thyroid function on the drugs, the risk of a sudden release of thyroid hormones is eliminated.

Most heart symptoms associated with hyperthyroidism disappear after treatment is successful. However, sometimes the atrial fibrillation does not reverse and may need continued treatment.

Checking Out Thyroid Nodules in Older People

Nodules are common in later life, but thyroid cancer is found less often in older than in younger people. The nodules are studied with a radioactive iodine scan to see whether or not they are active, and an ultrasound to see whether they are filled with fluid (cystic). Both of these characteristics point to a benign nodule rather than a cancer. Thyroid function tests can show whether the nodule is overactive and needs treatment.

In the final analysis, a fine needle aspiration biopsy is the best single test to rule out cancer in a nodule. If this test is positive for cancer, surgery is the treatment of choice, with follow-up similar to that for anyone with thyroid cancer (refer to Chapter 8).

Part V
The Part of Tens

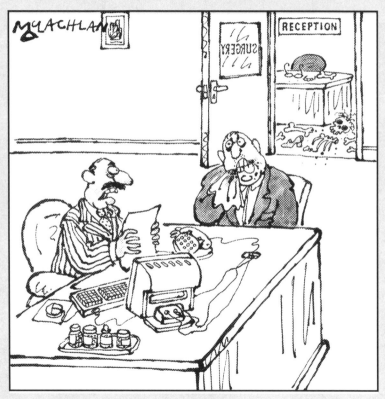

"Your bizarre eating disorder is due to a thyroid problem but that's no excuse for eating my receptionist, Mr. Weblott."

In this part . . .

As you would expect, a part of your body as important as the thyroid prompts all sorts of myths and mistaken ideas. Here you find the ones we consider the most important (and possibly the most damaging if you believe them). The final chapter shows you what you can do to make sure that you maximize your thyroid health in ten easy steps.

Chapter 21

Ten Myths about Thyroid Health

In This Chapter

▶ Getting the facts about weight loss and gain

▶ Learning the truth about hormone replacement

▶ Understanding how thyroid disease occurs

▶ Trusting your symptoms

*T*hanks to the Internet, you have access to incredible amounts of information about your thyroid. Unfortunately, a lot of the material is inaccurate, and importantly, you need to maintain a healthy degree of scepticism. This chapter aims to clear up some commonly held myths concerning the thyroid and its diseases.

I'm Hypothyroid, So I Can't Lose Weight

If you have hypothyroidism, or if you receive treatment for a thyroid condition and the cure results in an underactive thyroid, you may find you have a hard time losing weight. The myth is that you can't lose weight if you have hypothyroidism, even when it's properly treated. The truth is that a large percentage of people who are successfully treated for hypothyroidism weigh almost the same after treatment as they did before they developed the disease. And some people with hypothyroidism – mostly older people – actually lose weight, rather than gain it, after receiving replacement thyroid hormone. This loss occurs when a person is receiving poor nutrition, which is made worse with the general lack of interest that can accompany hypothyroidism, so the person is simply not interested in eating properly and consumes too few calories.

Keep in mind that hypothyroidism is associated with fatigue. Many people with hypothyroidism reduce their physical activity as a result and may not restore their previous level of activity after the hypothyroidism is treated properly.

If you struggle to lose any weight you've gained due to hypothyroidism, and if your activity level remains the same, it's possible that your thyroid treatment is inadequate (which is determined with a TSH test) or possibly that you need to take T3 replacement hormone in addition to T4 although this treatment is controversial (refer to Chapter 5).

You may also have another autoimmune condition present. Because the most common cause of hypothyroidism is autoimmune thyroiditis (refer to Chapter 5), ask your doctor to check you for diabetes mellitus Type 1 or auto-immune adrenal insufficiency (Addison's disease – failure to make the hormone cortisol), among other conditions. This check is easily done with a blood glucose test for diabetes or a serum cortisol level for autoimmune adrenal insufficiency.

The bottom line is that if you take in more energy (calories) than you need, you gain weight. If you take in too little energy, you lose weight. Another truth is that your metabolic rate declines, as does your tendency to move around, as you age. Both changes tend to make weight loss more difficult, but it's still possible.

If you have hypothyroidism and are on the proper dose of thyroid hormone, you can lose weight with sufficient diet and activity. So, try to eat less and exercise more. You may find that cutting back on your intake of refined carbo-hydrates (white bread, pasta, rice) and eating more wholegrain versions (brown bread, rice, and pasta) is helpful.

I'm Hyperthyroid, So I Can't Gain Weight

The myth that hyperthyroidism always causes weight loss is a source of confusion in making an accurate diagnosis. Although the majority of people do lose weight when they are hyperthyroid, some actually gain weight – especially the elderly.

A study published in the *Journal of the American Geriatric Society* in 1996, compared 19 classical signs of hyperthyroidism between older and younger patients. They found that three signs occur in more than 50 per cent of older people: rapid heartbeat, fatigue, and weight loss. However, some have no weight loss or even experience weight gain. Only two signs – loss of appetite and an irregular heart rhythm – happen more often in the older patients. Overall, of the 19 classical clinical signs, older people show only six of them on average, while younger people have 11.

Other studies show similar results and emphasise the importance of check-ing levels of thyroid hormones and TSH in older people before making a diag-nosis of hyperthyroidism.

Weight loss, as well as other symptoms of hyperthyroidism, is not always present. One solution is to get thyroid blood tests every five years, beginning at age 35, but costs of screening make this move controversial.

Breastfeeding and Antithyroid Pills Don't Mix

For years, doctors advised women taking antithyroid pills for hyperthyroidism during pregnancy not to breastfeed. This advice was in case medication entering the baby's circulation through the breast milk made the baby hypothyroid. This notion is now firmly in the realms of myth. Two important studies show this belief is incorrect. In one study published in the *Journal of Clinical Endocrinology and Metabolism*, 88 mothers took an antithyroid drug (methimazole, a drug similar to carbimazole that is in use in America) for 12 months. Close follow-up showed that all the babies of treated mothers had normal thyroid function. They grew normally, and had identical IQ, verbal, and functional tests to children who breast-fed from mothers without hyperthyroidism.

In a second study, breastfeeding mothers took another major antithyroid drug, propylthiouracil (PTU). Again the babies' had normal thyroid function tests and perfect development.

A hyperthyroid mother taking antithyroid drugs to control her hyperthyroidism may safely breastfeed her new baby.

Brand Name Thyroid Hormone Pills Are Best

The number of people taking thyroid replacement hormone throughout the world is enormous, and the amount of money spent on thyroid hormone replacement pills is also huge. The company that captures the largest share of the market makes its shareholders very happy.

A myth has arisen that cheaper, generic preparations of thyroxine (T4 hormone) are not equal in potency to brand name thyroxine. This myth began, as so many do, with research that was correct at the time but is now outdated. In a study published in the *Journal of the American Medical Association* in 1997, 20 women with hypothyroidism took four different preparations of T4, at the same dosage, for six weeks at a time, one after the other. Blood tests taken during this study show absolutely no difference in any of the preparations and all had equivalent activity. The preparations, including two brand names and two generics, are sufficiently equal in their activity that there is no reason to choose any one over the others. In the United Kingdom, most doctors prescribe generically, and most pharmacists dispense generically to help save the NHS money. You may find you get several different versions of T4 during your time on treatment, depending on which is available at the cheapest price. Generic thyroid preparations save the NHS money and are used interchangeably with brand name thyroxine.

I Have to Take Thyroid Medication for Life

Many patients believe that once they're on thyroid hormone replacement, they'll take it for life. For many people, this belief is true. Any treatment that removes or destroys much of the thyroid (such as surgery or radioactive iodine) does require treatment with thyroxine (T4 hormone) for life. However, in certain situations, hypothyroidism is temporary; you may need thyroxine for a time, but can later stop taking it. Sometimes, the fact that you no longer need the medication is obvious, but other times you and your doctor may decide to attempt a trial period off thyroid hormone for four to six weeks to see if you still need it.

The following are some of the conditions that require thyroid hormone replacement for a limited amount of time. Each is explained in detail in Chapter 11:

- ✔ *Subacute thyroiditis* causes the temporary breakdown of thyroid cells and the release of thyroxine from the thyroid. As this condition improves, thyroxine is made and stored again, and oral thyroxine is no longer necessary.

- ✔ *Silent and postpartum thyroiditis* also cause temporary loss of thyroxine, which is restored with time.

- ✔ *Acute thyroiditis* occasionally requires temporary treatment with thyroid hormone.

The major diagnosis that means you may or may not need to take thyroid hormone pills for life is chronic thyroiditis (also known as Hashimoto's or autoimmune thyroiditis – check out Chapter 5 for more on this condition). This condition is the result of antibodies that block TSH from sufficiently stimulating the thyroid to produce enough thyroid hormone. Occasionally, levels of blocking antibodies fall. The only way to know if this fall happens is to measure antibody levels or to stop the thyroid hormone and test thyroid function four to six weeks later. If your thyroid function remains normal, you may not need to take thyroxine any longer.

Depending on your diagnosis, you can sometimes stop taking thyroid hormone treatment at some point. It's well worth checking, particularly if you are less than 40 years of age.

Natural Thyroid Hormones Are Better Than Synthetic Hormones

The first thyroid hormones used to treat people with low thyroid function came from the thyroids of animals – a preparation called *desiccated thyroid* (refer to Chapter 5). After decades of use, desiccated thyroid is now replaced with synthetic thyroid hormones made in the laboratory. Some holdouts still believe desiccated thyroid is superior to synthetic thyroxine (T4 hormone) for treating hypothyroidism. As long ago as 1978, an article in the *American Journal of Medicine* asked 'Why does anyone still use desiccated thyroid?' The article declared desiccated thyroid an obsolete therapy.

Hormones extracted from animals have plenty of problems:

✔ Desiccated thyroid does not provide a standard amount from dose to dose because one animal has a different amount of hormones in its thyroid than the next animal.

✔ Not only does the dose of T4 and T3 in desiccated thyroid vary from pill to pill, but it does not provide the same levels as a normal thyroid releases.

✔ Desiccated thyroid contains animal impurities that can cause immune reactions.

✔ The use of desiccated thyroid confuses thyroid testing. If only the total T4 hormone is measured, that result is often low due to the large amount of T3 in the medication. The patient may receive even more thyroid hormone and actually become hyperthyroid.

The only thing going for desiccated thyroid is that it does contain some T3, which most synthetic hormone replacements do not. However, synthetic T3 does now exist, and is far superior to the mixture in desiccated thyroid.

Synthetic thyroxine is currently the medication of choice in the treatment of hypothyroidism. Some thyroid specialists believe that, in the future, treatment may advance to involve a combination of T4 and T3 in the exact ratio that it leaves the thyroid.

Thyroid Disease Is Catching

Understanding why this myth is so entrenched in the minds of the public isn't hard to do. Most thyroid disease is inherited; so the likelihood of finding the same disease in two sisters or a mother and her daughter is relatively high, suggesting that their physical closeness to one another causes one to catch the disease from the other. Furthermore, in areas where people don't consume enough iodine, practically everyone has thyroid disease – again suggesting that it's infectious.

Another situation that seems to suggest that thyroid disease is catching is the occurrence of thyroid disease after large-scale radiation exposure. Just about everyone comes down with some illness in that situation. Children, especially, often develop goitres, nodules, and thyroid cancers.

An understanding of the way these diseases develop, quickly clarifies the situation:

- ✔ Hereditary thyroid diseases affect the females of a family, usually sparing the males.
- ✔ After iodine is supplied, the incidence of thyroid disease rapidly declines in iodine-deficient areas.
- ✔ Children who take iodine pills or avoid exposure to radioactive iodine generally do not get thyroid diseases, while those who do not, will.
- ✔ You cannot catch thyroid disease, nor can you give it to someone else in the way that germs are passed from person to person.

Iodine Deficiency Is a Medical Problem

Because iodine deficiency (refer to Chapter 12) causes hypothyroidism, goitre, and cretinism (when severe), the belief that the disease responds to medical treatment with iodine seems clear-cut. If so, however, the disease would have disappeared years ago.

As with any major medical problem (like AIDS, breast cancer, and prostate cancer), iodine deficiency is a social, economic, and political problem as much as, or more than, it is a medical problem.

To begin with, an understanding about the cause of hypothyroidism in iodine-deficient areas is often lacking. The people are poor, work very hard, and have little time for the intricacies of the cause of disease. Their poverty means they cannot afford to pay for nurses to give them medication or inject them with iodised oil. They do not understand that certain foods, like cassava (a starchy tuberous root used to make flour), worsen the problem, so they continue to consume large quantities of them.

Often the local or national government pumps in lots of money to improve the situation and provides iodine supplementation, but provides no punishment for those who do not follow the regulations. Manufacturers may fail to put any iodine into their so-called 'iodised' salt and claim the subsidies for it anyway. Much of that money disappears after it leaves government control.

Sometimes, attempts to solve the problem run up against the realities of salt production – as is the case in Indonesia, for example, where salt is in the hands of numerous salt farmers rather than a centralised salt production facility (as in China). As a result, altering salt production to make enough iodised salt in China than in Indonesia is easier and more productive.

When there's a tremendous need for a substance like iodine, the cheats try to profit from people's misery. They charge more for iodised salt and then fail to actually iodise the salt. They also under price the government's iodised salt so that people buy their salt rather than true iodised salt from the government.

The instability of poor governments also plays a role. In Communist East Germany, iodine provision brought the disease under fairly good control. After the reunification of East and West Germany, however, the combined government neglected the problem and iodine deficiency started to reappear.

The solution to a clearly medical problem like iodine deficiency often involves social, cultural, and economic changes that populations resist, making a cure exceedingly difficult.

The Higher My Autoantibody Levels, the Worse My Thyroid Disease

This myth derives from a phenomenon that seems obvious: The more you have of something that denotes a disease, the worse that disease usually is. For example, if your temperature is 40 degrees Centigrade, you're probably sicker than someone whose temperature is only 38 degrees Centigrade. When it comes to thyroid autoantibodies, this notion isn't the case, however.

No correlation between levels of autoantibodies and the severity of someone's thyroid disease is apparent, however. Some of the sickest people with hyperthyroidism due to Graves' disease have relatively low levels of autoantibodies, while people with milder cases of Graves' may have high levels.

Adding to the confusion is the fact that thyroid autoantibodies often disappear after treatment with antithyroid drugs, and suggests the disease will not recur.

Also true is that very low levels of autoantibodies are often found in older women. But unless those women have abnormal thyroid function tests, the autoantibodies have little importance. Although people with low levels of autoantibodies are retested occasionally, they don't require treatment unless a thyroid condition develops.

And autoantibody levels are not comparable between laboratories. Little consistency stems from the methods used in the tests, so a level of 1,000 at one laboratory means something very different from a level of 1,000 at another laboratory.

Very high thyroid autoantibody levels do not indicate that you have a bad case of autoimmune thyroiditis. They simply confirm the diagnosis if other signs and symptoms exist.

Clinical Symptoms Are More Reliable Than Blood Tests

Thyroid disease is very confusing. In certain age groups, particularly older people, the expected signs and symptoms often do not exist. Sometimes, opposite symptoms are found. For example, some people gain weight as a result of hyperthyroidism, while others lose weight with hypothyroidism.

Many people, including some physicians, believe that clinical signs and symptoms are more accurate than laboratory tests when diagnosing thyroid conditions.

What would someone who relies on symptoms do with an older woman who is apathetic, does not have an enlarged thyroid, and is depressed, but has a high free T4 level and a low TSH? Her clinical signs and symptoms point to hypothyroidism, but her tests show hyperthyroidism. Relying on symptoms alone, a doctor might give this patient thyroid hormone replacement. The proof of the pudding is in the eating. When treating people with confusing clinical signs according to their lab test results rather than their clinical findings, they invariably get better.

One of the problems is that signs and symptoms of hypothyroidism are often very subtle, just like many other diseases. The signs and symptoms mimic those of diseases like depression, menopause, and ageing.

Another problem is the placebo effect of any drug. If you give a group of patients a drug that's not supposed to have any effect on the disease in question, a few of them will get better. This finding does not mean that the drug is the reason they improved.

A good physician bases his or her treatment on evidence-based medicine. This reasoning means that single instances of improvement do not prove that a treatment is correct; they could just as easily mean that the original diagnosis is wrong.

Do not take treatment for a thyroid disease, such as hyperthyroidism or hypothyroidism, unless your thyroid function tests confirm the diagnosis.

Chapter 22

Ten Ways to Maximise Thyroid Health

....

In This Chapter

▶ Keeping an eye out for thyroid disease

▶ Getting enough iodine

▶ Managing hyperthyroidism and cancer

▶ Avoiding drug interactions and radiation

▶ Staying up-to-date

....

*T*his book covers a lot of information. Now it's time to put the icing on the cake, or perhaps the exclamation point at the end of the sentence. This chapter discusses the steps you can take to ensure your best thyroid function. You may think there's little you can do – that your thyroid, like the River Thames, just keeps rolling along. Fortunately, that's not true – there's plenty you can do to maximise thyroid health.

These things fall into several categories. You can ensure that thyroid testing is done at the right intervals. You can examine yourself to determine whether the shape of your thyroid is normal. You can make sure that you're getting the proper nutrients so your thyroid makes its hormones in sufficient quantities. And perhaps most important of all, you can stay knowledgeable about all the new discoveries concerning thyroid health and disease that appear on a regular basis.

Carrying out these actions means you're doing all you can to take care of that little gland that weighs less than an ounce but which plays such an important role in your life and health.

Screening at Appropriate Intervals

Many symptoms of hypothyroidism are subtle or are similar to symptoms of ageing or menopause (refer to Chapter 5). Hyperthyroidism is also tricky as symptoms are not always prominent (especially in older people), and sometimes appear to point towards an underactive thyroid even though the thyroid is overactive, or the other way round (refer to Chapter 20).

The most common form of thyroid disease is autoimmune thyroiditis (also known as chronic thyroiditis or Hashimoto's thyroiditis). It probably affects 10 per cent of the population, although only a small fraction of people with this disease actually develop hypothyroidism.

Hypothyroidism often begins when a woman is in her 30s. For this reason, and because of the confusion that exists between the diagnosis and the signs and symptoms that a person experiences, some doctors suggest screening for abnormal thyroid function at age 35, continuing at five-year intervals for life. This course of action is fine if you can afford private health screening, but thyroid tests are usually only carried out in the NHS if symptoms, signs, or family history suggest that they're needed. Of course, if tests reveal a thyroid condition, free NHS testing is carried out as often as needed.

Screening involves having a blood test – the TSH (thyroid-stimulating hormone) test. The normal range, depending on the particular laboratory carrying out the test, is usually given as 0.3 to 4.5 µU/ml (microunits per millilitre) (check out Chapter 5). If your doctor tells you that your screening test is normal but you still have symptoms consistent with hypothyroidism, ask the doctor for the exact number of your TSH. If it's above 2.5, ask your doctor to consider giving you a trial of treatment with thyroid hormone replacement.

Checking Thyroid Function As Your Body Changes

If you're taking thyroid hormone treatment, you're on a fixed dose of medication. However, many physical states, particularly pregnancy (refer to Chapter 18), change the amount of thyroid hormone that you need to maintain normal function. The same is true as you get older.

Chemical changes that cause you to make more thyroid-binding proteins (check out Chapter 4) require you to take an increased dose of thyroid medication. Any condition that increases your oestrogen level is an example, such as pregnancy and taking the oral contraceptive pill. As more thyroid-binding protein is made, more of your dose of thyroid binds to the protein and less is available to enter your cells. You must increase your dose of thyroid hormone. Blood tests determine when you again have enough.

Chemical changes that cause you to make less thyroid-binding protein require a decreased dose of thyroid hormone. If you take androgens (refer to Chapter 10) or have a disease that causes excessive production of androgens, you may need your dosage of thyroid hormone reduced. Less thyroid-binding protein means less binding of your thyroid dose, so more is available to enter cells. If you don't reduce your dose of thyroid hormone in this circumstance, you could become hyperthyroid.

Another situation that occurs in pregnancy is the reduction in autoimmunity (refer to Chapter 18). If you're treating hyperthyroidism with antithyroid pills, you may need a lower dose or none at all until the pregnancy is completed. Then you will need treatment again.

During times of major body change such as pregnancy or illness, your need for thyroid hormone or antithyroid medication may change. The only way to know that you're on the right dose is to have thyroid function tests at regular intervals, usually every three months.

Performing a 'Neck Check'

Five steps are involved in doing a 'Neck Check'. You need a hand-held mirror and a glass of water. The steps are:

1. **Hold the mirror in your hand, focusing on the area of your neck just below your Adam's apple and immediately above your collarbone.** Your thyroid is located in this area of your neck.

2. **While focusing on this area in the mirror, tip your head back.**

3. **Take a drink of water and swallow.**

4. **As you swallow, look at your neck. Check for any bulges or protrusions in this area when you swallow.** Reminder: Don't confuse your Adam's apple with the thyroid gland. The thyroid gland is located farther down on your neck, closer to the collarbone. You may want to repeat this process several times.

5. **If you do see any bulges or protrusions in this area, see your doctor.** You may have an enlarged thyroid gland or a thyroid nodule that needs checking to determine whether cancer is present or if treatment for thyroid disease is needed.

You can detect abnormalities in the size and shape of your thyroid gland. If you think your thyroid is enlarged, see your doctor to determine if there's any problem.

Getting Enough Iodine to Satisfy Your Thyroid

The number of people with iodine deficiency in Europe is on the increase. Many people do not eat good food sources of iodine, namely fish and, to a lesser extent, meat, eggs, and milk, and there's a little iodine in fruits and vegetables, too.

Due to concerns about high blood pressure, your doctor may urge you to cut back on salt intake as salt raises blood pressure. Recommendations are to limit salt intake to less than 6 grams daily, slightly more than a teaspoon. This reduced amount contains plenty of iodine for your diet however, as 1 teaspoon of salt contains about 400 micrograms of iodine. Or you can eat a couple slices of bread each day. Each slice of bread contains about 150 micrograms of iodine. The recommended daily intake of iodine is 150 to 200 micrograms.

Stopping Thyroid Medication, If Possible

Some people who take thyroid hormone replacement because of laboratory evidence of low thyroid function can stop their treatment at some point. These people have hypothyroidism due to chronic thyroiditis (refer to Chapter 5). Their hypothyroidism is the result of antibodies that block the action of thyroid-stimulating hormone. Up to 25 per cent of these patients can come off treatment as, over time, the level of their blocking antibodies may fall to the point that their thyroid gland is able to make its own thyroid hormone. It's certainly worth trying to stop thyroid hormone after a few years of treatment to see if the thyroid can function on its own.

If you have hypothyroidism due to chronic thyroiditis and have taken thyroid hormone pills for a few years, ask your doctor if you can stop the thyroid hormone replacement for a month and check your thyroid function tests.

Using Both Types of Thyroid Hormone

The thyroid gland makes two different thyroid hormones, T4, the major component, and T3, which is the active form of thyroid hormone but made in much lower amounts in the gland (check out Chapter 3).

Because drug manufacturers learned to synthesise it, T4 is the only treatment prescribed when people need thyroid hormone. It's given so that a patient's

TSH level returns to normal, as does the free T4 in the blood. This practise means that most people who are treated for hypothyroidism have a deficiency of T3.

In practical terms, this problem is not significant. However, a few people continue to complain of symptoms of low thyroid function despite normal laboratory test results. These patients may improve if T3 is added to their treatment.

Doctors find that measuring this kind of improvement objectively is difficult because the test results remain in the normal range. Monitoring relies on the subjective symptoms of the patient indicating that he or she feels better on the combination therapy compared to T4 alone.

This from of treatment is still a grey area in medicine as randomised controlled trials have not yet shown definite benefit from giving both T3 and T4. If you have symptoms of hypothyroidism and are taking T4 hormone replacement alone, ask your doctor to investigate the possibility of prescribing a small dose of T3 as you may do better with the combination.

Preventing the Regrowth of Thyroid Cancer

If you have thyroid cancer, you've probably had thyroid surgery followed with irradiation to eliminate the remaining thyroid tissue. Now you want to prevent any regrowth of thyroid cancer. This prevention is accomplished with sufficient thyroid hormone to suppress the production of thyroid-stimulating hormone – meaning the goal is for your TSH level to drop below the normal range. The lower level of the normal range is usually 0.3 µU/ml (microunits per millilitre) although laboratories can vary, so you generally want a reading of 0.3 or below to ensure your thyroid isn't stimulated.

But how low is too low? If a reading of 0.3 is good, is a reading of 0.1 better? A study published in *Thyroid* in 1999, addressed this issue. The researchers had two groups of cancer patients: in one group, TSH levels were suppressed to below 0.1; in the other group TSH levels were kept between 0.4 and 0.1. The study found that residual thyroid tissue was no more suppressed when the TSH was less than 0.1 than when it was less than 0.4. The research shows that thyroid cancer patients should receive suppressive doses of T4 but that greater suppression is no better than lesser degrees of suppression.

The advantage of taking the least suppressive dose of thyroid hormone possible is that you have less risk of developing osteoporosis or rapid heartbeats, particularly if you are middle-aged or older.

Anticipating Drug Interactions

So many drugs interact with thyroid hormones that you must check with your doctor whenever you are placed on a new medication or taken off an old medication (look at Chapter 10).

Thyroid function is often affected not only when you start a new medication, but also if you are taken off an old medication or the dosage is changed significantly.

The way to avoid a problem is to perform (or ask your doctor or pharmacist to perform) a search for interactions between thyroid hormone and the drugs you need to take.

Drugs can affect thyroid function at any level. They can increase or decrease the release of thyrotrophin-releasing hormone, which affects how much thyroid-stimulating hormone (TSH) your body makes. They can increase or decrease the release of thyroid hormone from the thyroid. They can change the ratio of T4 hormone versus T3. They can affect the uptake of thyroid hormone into cells. They can increase or decrease the action of thyroid hormone within the cells.

The major drugs to take care with are the following (refer to Chapter 10):

- Amiodarone
- Aspirin (in doses greater than 3,000 milligrams)
- Corticosteroids
- Iodine
- Iron tablets
- Lithium
- Oestrogen
- Propranolol

Chances are that you will take one or more of these drugs in your lifetime.

Just about every drug affects thyroid function in one way or another. Fortunately, most of the effects are overcome as the normal thyroid gland makes some adjustment. But if you're on a fixed treatment dose of thyroid hormone, your thyroid cannot adjust as it would normally. Ask your doctor about having your thyroid function tested four to six weeks after you start a new medication or stop an old one.

Protecting Your Thyroid from Radiation

Between 1920 and 1960, many people received irradiation treatment that increases their risk for thyroid cancer. Close to 10 per cent of people receiving this treatment have developed thyroid cancer to date.

If you received irradiation to your neck area as a child because of enlarged tonsils, acne, an enlarged thymus, or some other condition, you are at increased risk for thyroid cancer and should inform your doctor. And if you've had any kind of radiation treatment to your head, chest, or neck in the past, it's important to perform the 'Neck Check' described earlier in this chapter. If you feel something unusual in your thyroid shape or size, see your doctor. In fact, see your doctor anyway as changes are often subtle and the incidence of thyroid cancer is definitely higher if you've had irradiation therapy. The exception here is that radiation treatment for hyperthyroidism does not increase your risk of cancer.

A thyroid scan or a thyroid ultrasound (check out Chapter 4) usually finds any significant abnormality that exists. If one is found, the usual next step is a fine needle biopsy of the thyroid.

What about follow-up if nothing is found? It's probably a good idea to have an examination of your thyroid on at least an annual basis if you have a history of thyroid exposure to radiation (other than for treatment for hyperthyroidism). However, should cancer occur, it's no more dangerous than thyroid cancer not associated with radiation, as long as it's treated properly.

Keeping Up-to-Date with Thyroid Discoveries

This book is an excellent start in your quest for knowledge about the thyroid gland and how it affects you. Given the pace of research, however, a book cannot keep you completely up-to-date with new findings about the thyroid gland. You need to seek them out for yourself. Where do you look?

In Appendix B, you find the Internet sites that are most accurate and reliable with respect to thyroid function and disease. These include Web sites of large organisations, sites belonging to individuals and groups who are advocates for various thyroid conditions, and government sites that provide information about the thyroid.

Drug companies that make thyroid medications have Web sites that contain information about their products and often general information about the thyroid as well.

Part VI
Appendixes

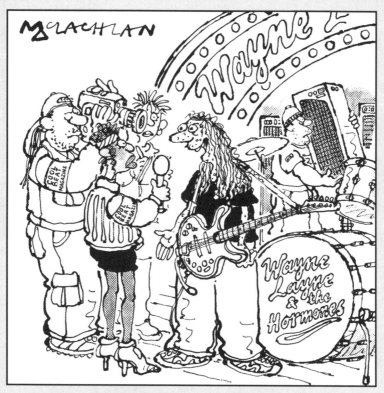

"Bad skin, lifeless hair, hoarse voice, loss of hearing—Thyroid disease has done wonders for my pop music career."

In this part . . .

Appendix A is a glossary of the terms you encounter as you read and hear about the thyroid gland, its function, and its diseases. All the strange words you meet for the first time in the text of the book are listed here and defined. Appendix B shows you where to look for more information as well as the latest research findings on the thyroid. There is a huge amount of research focusing on every aspect of normal thyroid function and abnormal thyroid conditions. This book gives you a good working knowledge of the subject, but there is always more to know, and these Web sites are where to find it.

Appendix A

A Glossary of Key Terms

Acute thyroiditis: A sudden-onset bacterial or fungal infection of the thyroid.

Allele: One of two or more genes that determine which enzyme is made or which body characteristic prevails.

Antigen: A foreign protein that prompts the production of antibodies to destroy it.

Autoimmune thyroiditis: Inflammation of the thyroid associated with the production of antibodies against thyroid tissue – also known as Hashimoto's thyroiditis or chronic thyroiditis.

Beta-blocking agent: One of a group of drugs given to block some of the adverse effects of excess thyroid hormone.

Chromosome: One of 23 pairs in the nucleus of every human cell that carry all the genes that determine the characteristics of the body.

Chronic thyroiditis: Another name for autoimmune thyroiditis.

Cretinism: A syndrome affecting children; its most outstanding feature is mental retardation that results from a lack of iodine during pregnancy.

Cyst: A sac-like structure containing fluid.

Dominant gene: The gene that determines which particular enzyme or body characteristic is expressed when two different genes are present.

Ectopic thyroid: Thyroid tissue found in an abnormal site, such as the base of the tongue.

Exophthalmos: Eye disease associated with Graves' disease.

Fine needle aspiration biopsy (FNAB): The process of putting a tiny needle into tissue, in this case the thyroid, for the purpose of determining the nature of that tissue. This process is particularly helpful for identifying thyroid cancer.

Free thyroxine (FT4): The tiny fraction of the T4 hormone that is not bound to protein and is therefore available to enter cells.

Free thyroxine index (FTI): An obsolete test once used to determine thyroid function. The product of multiplying the total T4 by the T3 resin uptake.

Free triiodothyronine (FT3): The tiny fraction of the T3 hormone that is not bound to protein and is therefore available to enter cells.

Gestational transient thyrotoxicosis: A brief period of hyperthyroidism during pregnancy that results from the large production of human chorionic gonadotrophin (which acts as a thyroid stimulator).

Goitre: An enlarged thyroid gland.

Graves' disease: An autoimmune condition that combines hyperthyroidism, eye disease, and skin disease.

Hashimoto's thyroiditis: Another name for autoimmune or chronic thyroiditis.

Heterozygous: Possessing two different genes for an enzyme or trait.

Homozygous: Possessing two of the same gene for an enzyme or trait.

Human chorionic gonadotrophin (HCG): A hormone made in the placenta that shares some properties with thyroid-stimulating hormone.

Hyperthyroidism: An over-active state due to the excessive production or intake of thyroid hormone.

Hypothyroidism: An under-active state due to the diminished production or intake of thyroid hormone.

Isthmus of the thyroid: The thyroid tissue that connects both lobes of the thyroid.

Leptin: A hormone produced in fat cells that signals the brain that the intake of calories is excessive.

Levothyroxine: The generic name for thyroxine (T4) medication.

Liothyronine: The generic name for triiodothyronine (T3) medication.

Medullary thyroid cancer: A cancer in the thyroid associated with cells called parafollicular or C-cells, which make a hormone called calcitonin.

Multinodular goitre: An enlargement of the thyroid associated with many nodules or outgrowths.

Multiple endocrine neoplasia (MEN): Hereditary production of tumours in several endocrine glands – one of the types of tumour is medullary thyroid cancer.

Mutation: An unexpected change in an enzyme or body characteristic due to an alteration in a particular gene.

Myxoedema: Another name for hypothyroidism.

Postpartum thyroiditis: Inflammation of the thyroid, after a pregnancy, that is associated with thyroid autoantibodies and may go through stages of hyperthyroidism, normal thyroid function, and hypothyroidism. It may resolve or end in hypothyroidism. It is often accompanied with depression.

Pyramidal lobe of the thyroid: An accessory lobe rising from the isthmus of the thyroid.

Recessive gene: A gene that determines an enzyme or body characteristic only when it is present on both chromosomes. (Otherwise the dominant gene prevails.)

Resin T3 uptake: A test of thyroid function (now obsolete) that provides an assessment of the amount of T4 bound to protein compared to the free T4.

Riedel's thyroiditis: A rare form of thyroid inflammation that is often associated with thyroid antibodies. It results in fibrosis of thyroid tissue, and sometimes parathyroid tissue, with tight adherence to the trachea.

Silent thyroiditis: A form of thyroiditis that is identical to postpartum thyroiditis but occurs at any time of life.

Subacute thyroiditis: A viral inflammation of the thyroid gland that is associated with pain in the thyroid.

Subclinical hypothyroidism: An elevation of the TSH, with a normal free T4 level and minimal to no symptoms of hypothyroidism.

Thiocyanate: A chemical found in some foods that may interfere with thyroid function.

Thyroglobulin: Material in the follicle of the thyroid in which thyroid hormones are stored.

Thyroid agenesis: Developmental failure to produce a thyroid gland in the foetus.

Thyroid autoantibodies: Proteins that react against the thyroid, sometimes to suppress or destroy it and sometimes to stimulate it.

Thyroid dysgenesis: Failure of the thyroid to grow or move into its proper place in the neck (attached to the trachea below the Adam's apple).

Thyroid hypoplasia: Production of a thyroid gland that is inadequate for the needs of the body.

Thyroid scan and uptake: Use of radioactive iodine to outline the thyroid, determine if tissue is actively producing thyroid hormone, and determine the level of activity of the gland.

Thyroid-stimulating hormone (TSH): A hormone from the pituitary gland that stimulates the thyroid to produce more hormone.

Thyroid storm: A very severe form of hyperthyroidism with high fever and severe sickness. It is a medical emergency.

Thyroid ultrasound: Use of sound waves to outline the thyroid and determine if growths are solid or cystic.

Thyrotrophin-releasing hormone (TRH): A hormone from the hypothalamus in the brain that stimulates the production and release of thyroid hormone through thyroid-stimulating hormone (TSH).

Thyroxine (T4): The major thyroid hormone.

Thyroxine-binding protein: Several proteins that bind the T3 and T4 hormones, making them unavailable to enter cells.

Total thyroxine: The sum of the thyroxine bound and unbound to thyroid-binding proteins.

Transient congenital hypothyroidism: Temporary hypothyroidism in newborns that often results from prematurity.

Triiodothyronine (T3): The active form of thyroid hormone.

Vitiligo: Patchy loss of skin pigment sometimes found in autoimmune diseases.

Appendix B

Sources of More Information

• •

*T*his appendix describes Web sites that offer information on thyroid disease, thyroid research, specialists in the field of thyroid health and disease. Many of the sites point to other links that provide still more information.

You can generally depend upon the information in these sites. But no matter what you read online, never make changes in your thyroid care without consulting your physician.

British Thyroid Association: www.british-thyroid-association.org. The British Thyroid Association is a learned society of clinical specialists involved in treating thyroid diseases. The Web site contains some useful information for patients.

British Thyroid Foundation: www.btf-thyroid.org. The British Thyroid Foundation is a charity that works together with the medical profession to support patients with thyroid conditions, and to raise money for thyroid research.

European Thyroid Association: www.eurothyroid.com. This organisation of European thyroid specialists promotes research and education about thyroid disease.

Mayo Clinic Foundation for Medical Education and Research: www.mayoclinic.com. This site is an excellent source of patient information on major thyroid conditions.

Medline Plus Thyroid Diseases: www.nlm.nih.gov/medlineplus/thyroiddiseases.html. This service of the National Library of Medicine provides information about thyroid disease management and research.

Merck Thyrolink: www.thyrolink.com. This service of Merck Pharmaceutical Company offers patient information in English, German, and French.

NHS Direct Online: www.nhsdirect.nhs.uk. The NHS on-line site that provides information on common health conditions, including thyroid problems.

Online Mendelian Inheritance in Man: www.ncbi.nlm.nih.gov/Omim. This site is a huge database of diseases that are inherited by getting a single gene. If you search by 'thyroid', you find all the currently known thyroid disorders in this database.

Patients Association: www.patients-association.org.uk. A charity that helps patients raise concerns and share experiences of healthcare.

Prodigy Knowledge: www.prodigy.nhs.uk. Prodigy Knowledge is an up-to-date NHS source of information for healthcare professionals and patients. It provides information on over 200 common conditions, including hyperthyroidism and hyperthyroidism.

Thyroid Cancer Support UK: www.thyroidcancersupportuk.org. This is a Yahoo support network and chat group for people with thyroid cancer. It is a forum in which people are able to support and encourage each other and to share experiences of diagnosis, operations, and the effects of treatment.

Thyroid Cancer Support Group – Wales: www.thyroidsupportwales.co.uk. A small support group for people with thyroid cancer who live in South Wales.

Thyroid Eye Disease Surgery Information: www.eyelidsurgery.co.uk. The Web site of an eye surgeon that provides information on the types of surgery available to treat thyroid eye disease.

Thyroid Eye Disease Charitable Trust: www.tedct.co.uk. Information from a charity that provides information and support for people with thyroid eye disease.

Thyroid Federation International: www.thyroid-fed.org. This organisation was founded in 1995 to deal with the problems of thyroid disease on a global basis. It's mainly involved in helping people start a thyroid patient organisation in their country or locale.

Index

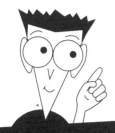

FOR DUMMIES®

Do Anything. Just Add Dummies

HOME

UK editions

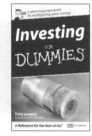

0-7645-7027-7

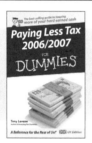

0-470-02921-8

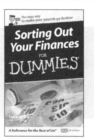

0-7645-7054-4

PERSONAL FINANCE

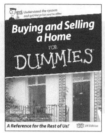

0-7645-7023-4

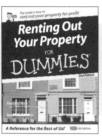

0-470-02860-2

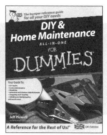

0-7645-7039-0

BUSINESS

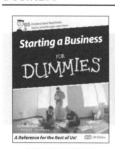

0-7645-7018-8

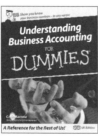

0-7645-7025-0

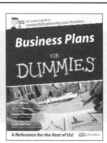

0-7645-7026-9

Answering Tough Interview Questions For Dummies (0-470-01903-4)

Arthritis For Dummies (0-470-02582-4)

Being the Best Man For Dummies (0-470-02657-X)

British History For Dummies (0-7645-7021-8)

Building Confidence For Dummies (0-470-01669-8)

Buying a Home on a Budget For Dummies (0-7645-7035-8)

Buying a Property in Eastern Europe For Dummies (0-7645-7047-1)

Children's Health For Dummies (0-470-02735-5)

Cognitive Behavioural Therapy For Dummies (0-470-01838-0)

CVs For Dummies (0-7645-7017-X)

Diabetes For Dummies (0-7645-7019-6)

Divorce For Dummies (0-7645-7030-7)

eBay.co.uk For Dummies (0-7645-7059-5)

European History For Dummies (0-7645-7060-9)

Gardening For Dummies (0-470-01843-7)

Golf For Dummies (0-470-01811-9)

Hypnotherapy For Dummies (0-470-01930-1)

Irish History For Dummies (0-7645-7040-4)

Marketing For Dummies (0-7645-7056-0)

Neuro-linguistic Programming For Dummies (0-7645-7028-5)

Nutrition For Dummies (0-7645-7058-7)

Parenting For Dummies (0-470-02714-2)

Pregnancy For Dummies (0-7645-7042-0)

Retiring Wealthy For Dummies (0-470-02632-4)

Rugby Union For Dummies (0-470-03537-4)

Small Business Employment Law For Dummies (0-7645-7052-8)

Starting a Business on eBay.co.uk For Dummies (0-470-02666-9)

Su Doku For Dummies (0-470-01892-5)

The GL Diet For Dummies (0-470-02753-3)

UK Law and Your Rights For Dummies (0-470-02796-7)

Wills, Probate and Inheritance Tax For Dummies (0-7645-7055-2)

Winning on Betfair For Dummies (0-470-02856-4)

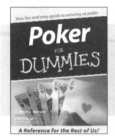 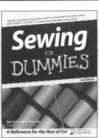 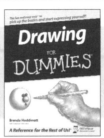
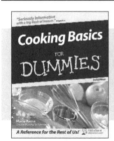 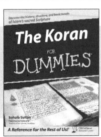 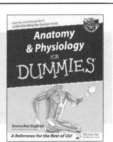
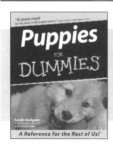 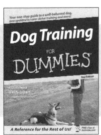 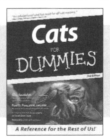

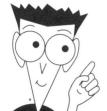

FOR DUMMIES®

The easy way to get more done and have more fun

LANGUAGES

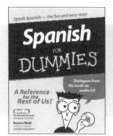

0-7645-5194-9

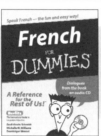

0-7645-5193-0

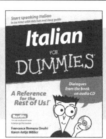

0-7645-5196-5

Also available:

Chinese For Dummies
(0-471-78897-X)

Chinese Phrases
For Dummies
(0-7645-8477-4)

French Phrases For Dummies
(0-7645-7202-4)

German For Dummies
(0-7645-5195-7)

Italian Phrases For Dummies
(0-7645-7203-2)

Japanese For Dummies
(0-7645-5429-8)

Latin For Dummies
(0-7645-5431-X)

Spanish Phrases
For Dummies
(0-7645-7204-0)

Spanish Verbs For Dummies
(0-471-76872-3)

Hebrew For Dummies
(0-7645-5489-1)

MUSIC AND FILM

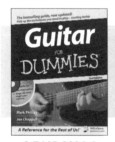

0-7645-9904-6

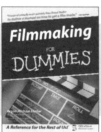

0-7645-2476-3

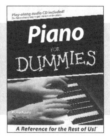

0-7645-5105-1

Also available:

Bass Guitar For Dummies
(0-7645-2487-9)

Blues For Dummies
(0-7645-5080-2)

Classical Music For Dummies
(0-7645-5009-8)

Drums For Dummies
(0-471-79411-2)

Jazz For Dummies
(0-471-76844-8)

Opera For Dummies
(0-7645-5010-1)

Rock Guitar For Dummies
(0-7645-5356-9)

Screenwriting For Dummies
(0-7645-5486-7)

Songwriting For Dummies
(0-7645-5404-2)

Singing For Dummies
(0-7645-2475-5)

HEALTH, SPORTS & FITNESS

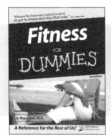

0-7645-7851-0

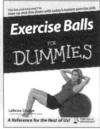

0-7645-5623-1

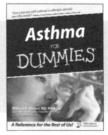

0-7645-4233-8

Also available:

Controlling Cholesterol
For Dummies
(0-7645-5440-9)

Dieting For Dummies
(0-7645-4149-8)

High Blood Pressure
For Dummies
(0-7645-5424-7)

Martial Arts For Dummies
(0-7645-5358-5)

Menopause For Dummies
(0-7645-5458-1)

Power Yoga For Dummies
(0-7645-5342-9)

Weight Training
For Dummies
(0-471-76845-6)

Yoga For Dummies
(0-7645-5117-5)

9160_p3

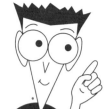
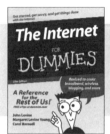
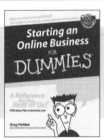
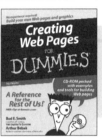
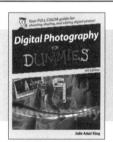
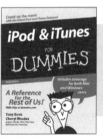
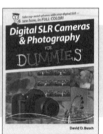
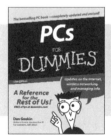
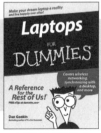
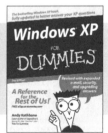